A Long Way from Henry Street

A Collection of Stories Written by

School Nurses

MACGILL

Discount School Nurse Supplies

Compiled and Edited by Matt Flesch

Assistant Editors:
Nick Heidtbrink
Therese Hanlon
Kimberly Pinter

Front Cover Art by Mike Schmidt
Back Cover Photography of the Henry Street Settlement by Jessica Tagliaferro

MacGill & Company
1000 North Lombard Road
Lombard, IL 60148
800-323-2841
www.macgill.com

First Edition

ISBN 0-9744720-0-X

Contents

Introduction

At the end of the 19th century, the Lower East Side of New York City was an impoverished neighborhood with cramped living spaces—which translated to dismal public health conditions.

Lilliam Wald, a student at the Women's Medical College of New York, refused to accept the living conditions of this neighborhood and set out on a lifelong mission to make healthcare services more accessible. Her vision of "public health nursing" led to the building of the Henry Street Settlement which provided health services to the people of New York's Lower East Side. Continuing her vision of public health, Wald placed a nurse from the Henry Street Settlement, Lina Rogers Struthers, at a public school to reduce absenteeism and the spread of communicable diseases among children. Struthers was so successful that the New York City Board of Health organized a public school nursing program, the first such service offered anywhere in the world.

One-hundred years later, over 50,000 school nurses nationwide bring the same core values to their jobs as Struthers did in 1902. Since the days when Henry Street nurses tended to children's needs, however, much has changed. *A Long Way from Henry Street* brings light to the changing role of school nurses and the new challenges that face them in today's society.

The stories in this book were written by school nurses who work in a diverse range of environments. From small Midwestern towns to large coastal cities—impoverished inner-city neighborhoods to wealthy suburbs—these stories focus on a wide range of challenges and experiences that school nurses encounter.

There are stories that reveal how school nurses confronted healthcare providers to ensure that a child received accurate diagnosis and treatment, often bringing a family medical care that was otherwise unattainable. Other stories show how nurses were able to look beyond a child's physical pain and offer much needed emotional support and guidance. Stories that chronicle the typical chaotic day in the life of a school nurse are included as well as instances where school nurses helped students overcome personal trauma. Of course, no book focusing on school nursing would be complete without humorous stories. This book contains more than one story about the innocent behavior of children that will make you laugh.

We encourage you to pass this book on to those who may not be aware of the need for school nurses and the impact they have on children's health. There are still many who don't realize that our changing society has brought about a whole new job description for school nurses. An increasing number of kids go to school with significant handicaps, chronic illness, and from troubled homes. Judith Dorward, RN, poignantly describes the changing needs of children in her story entitled *The Clinic*: "The 1950's are over. Donna Reed is not waiting at home with cookies and milk. She is divorced and working while trying to go to school so that someday she can get a job with benefits. Her kids have very real needs that can be addressed by caring and imaginative people who are at school often enough to be available to children."

A Long Way from Henry Street is written by and about the caring and imaginative school nurses who devote their lives to keeping children healthy and happy.

Confidentiality

Great measures were taken to ensure that strict confidentiality is maintained in each of the stories included in this book. Stories were reviewed and given special attention if they revealed private information about any individual. The names of students, parents, physicians and other parties have been changed or omitted in the vast majority of stories. Further, any references to the names of schools, streets, cities and states were omitted when necessary. In some cases, the name of the author of a story was omitted to be certain that no correlation could be made between a student and a personal situation. In other instances, even despite the fact that real names were not used, the author and/or editor sought and received permission to print from individuals described in their story.

Request for Feedback

We hope you enjoy this collection of stories and appreciate any feedback you might have. Please send your comments via email to macgill@macgill.com or by regular mail to MacGill & Company, 1000 North Lombard Road, Lombard, IL, 60148. Your feedback will help us determine whether to publish a second edition of *A Long Way from Henry Street* .

If you are interested in submitting a story for publication in potential future editions of *A Long Way from Henry Street*, please visit www.macgill.com for submission guidelines.

Acknowledgements

MacGill & Company would like to thank all of the school nurses who took time out of their busy schedules to submit a story for inclusion in this book. The sheer number of submissions that we received outnumbered the amount of pages we were able to print, regretfully forcing us to leave out many excellent stories.

We also thank the National Association of School Nurses (NASN), its state affiliates and the National Association of State School Nurse Consultants for spreading the word about this book during its initial stages of production. In particular, we would like to thank the following people for their guidance and/or contributions:

NASN President Janice Hootman, PhD, RN, BSN, MS

Linda Davis-Alldritt, MA, PHN, RN

Caroline E. Green, BSN, CHES, RN

Victoria Jackson, MS, RN, NCSN

Dorothy Marks, RN

DeEtte Hall, MSN, RN

Patricia Clemen, MTS, BSN, RN

Donna Mazyck, BSN, RN, NCSN

Therese Hanlon

Judy Watson, RN

Mary Ann Phillips, RN

Kimberly Pinter

Finally, we would like to express our gratitude to the Henry Street Settlement for providing the photography featured on the back cover of this book. The Henry Street Settlement is located in New York, NY. Its core mission is to challenge the effects of urban poverty by providing individuals and families with essential social and cultural services. More information regarding the Henry Street Settlement can be found at www.henrystreet.org.

I

Advocating for Children's Health

"Our job as certified school nurses is to be advocates for the children in our care. When neither the child nor their parents are able to speak up, we need to do it for them."

—Caroline Champion, RN, MSN, CSN

Out of Darkness

By Kimberly Toole, RN, MSN

As supervisor of a school nursing program and a former school nurse, I am fortunate to work with some of the finest school nurses in the country. Within the public school district that employs me, I hear about or witness extraordinary feats of compassion and mercy on a daily basis. The following is a story about a nurse named Linda who has gone well beyond the call of duty on behalf of children.

Linda is a school nurse at an inner-city elementary school with an overall poverty level of 90–100 percent. The children she serves usually come to school with a whole array of problems and Linda always considers the whole child. She considers not only their physical complaint or ailment, but also what may be going on at home with the rest of their family. The school's principal once said, "Linda practices holistic nursing, always considering the child's physical, emotional and psychological well-being, as well as their academic success." I couldn't say it better.

A couple of years ago, a child moved to this city with his mother, two older siblings, his grandmother, his aunt and his uncle. The grandmother was the head of the household, but was morbidly obese, very ill and unable to leave her home. She ruled the family from a bed, was very argumentative and difficult to communicate with. Nobody could convince her to obtain medical care for herself or the children. She and the other adults in the family were illiterate, mentally challenged, very low functioning and very suspicious of outsiders. With extreme patience

Linda gradually developed rapport with the family and was finally let into their home.

While the older siblings were enrolled in school, the youngest child was kept at home. He was extremely hyperactive with dysmorphic features and was not potty-trained. He was ill kept and seemingly alienated. It was evident that the family treated this child differently than the others. During Linda's home visits, the child sat alone in a dark back room. Very concerned with this situation, Linda contacted children's services with the hope of bringing the child aid. When help was declined because the child's situation was not considered severe enough neglect, Linda decided to take matters into her own hands.

Linda convinced the family to allow her to enroll the child in kindergarten. She managed to find a developmentally handicapped classroom for him, which happened to have a very loving and patient teacher. Linda also assisted in getting the child a wrap-around instructional assistant for one-on-one assistance with toileting and hygiene. Because of their carefull planning and guidance the child grew to love school and really blossomed. He was still not treated right at home, but always looked forward to going to school. School was his "safe haven," and he knew he could always count on his teacher or his school nurse, Linda.

Linda also made referrals to the Bureau for Children with Medical Handicaps (BCMH) so that the child could get a thorough diagnostic evaluation from both a genetics clinic and a pediatric gastroenterologist. The geneticist said that the child should have been seen years ago and found that he had a rare genetic disorder. Linda also made sure that the child had regular care at a nearby health center. Although he had lice and toilet accidents, she drove him and his mother to all of his appointments and served as interpreter for the mother. The physician put the child on medication, which helped his hyperactivity and behavioral problems. Linda also helped the family apply and obtain public assistance, medical coverage, homemaker services, and services from the Department of Mental Retardation and Developmental Disabilities (MRDD). Since the family was illiterate and distrusting of strangers, all appointments, applications, information, and other paperwork had to go through Linda or the mother would not follow through. Linda made numerous home visits and even helped the entire family eradicate lice.

She also helped one of the siblings who had chronic throat infections, enlarged tonsils, and sleep apnea by applying to BCMH so he could have a needed tonsillectomy and adenoidectomy.

Linda gave this family, like others, her all. It is difficult to say what would have happened to this family, especially the youngest child, if Linda hadn't intervened and been his advocate in almost every aspect of his life. If not for Linda, he may still be sitting in a dark corner somewhere in his grandmother's apartment.

To contact Kimberly Toole, send an email to macgill@macgill.com.

Under the Wings of Care

By Caroline Champion, RN, MSN, CSN

During mid-September of my fifth year as a certified school nurse a new student who was educable handicapped (EMH) and whose family was poor and uneducated suffered a grand mal seizure on the playground. When her teacher and aide brought her into my office, she was still seizing and was not breathing. Her lip color quickly changed to blue and her skin became dusky. I immediately began rescue breathing and told the teacher to call 911. Her seizure started slowing and she began breathing on her own. In the time it took the ambulance to arrive, she seized two more times, and each time I had to breathe for her. At my principal's request, I accompanied her in the ambulance on the way to the ER. She did not seize again while at the hospital and I returned to school soon after her mother arrived.

That evening, her mother called and said that the hospital released the child shortly after I left with no instructions, no medication and no follow-up but left a hep-loc (a device to administer IV fluids) in her arm. I walked the mother through the process of removing the device on the phone. The child was back at school the following day.

Almost a week to the day, the child began seizing again—this time in the classroom. I was called to the room and a familiar scene evolved. She had stopped breathing and I again had to breathe for her. We called 911 and since we had had a bad experience at the first hospital, I suggested that the child be taken to the other one in town. At my request, my principal called his child's pediatrician who agreed to being involved in the child's care. This time we figured everything had been covered to give this child the best possible care.

The child had a grand mal seizure upon arrival at the ER which was observed by a doctor. He admitted her and called the pediatrician. Again, after the mother arrived, I left. I felt assured that this time the child would be taken care of properly. How naive I was!

This second episode happened on a Friday. On Sunday, I received a phone call from the child's mother saying her daughter had been released. Like before, she was sent home with no instructions, no medication, and no diagnosis. Fortunately, she did not come home with a hep-loc.

On Monday morning I called the child's pediatrician and got a reply and attitude toward the case that was unbelievable. He said the nurses on the pediatric floor reported that the child was faking seizures. Then he added, "Even if she has epilepsy, how is her mother going to take care of her? She (the mother) has a mentality even lower than the child."

He arrived at this conclusion despite the fact that an EEG (a brain wave to test for epilepsy) had not been performed. I attempted to explain to him that the child had an IQ of 70 or lower and would not have the intelligence to fake a seizure. Trying to stay calm—and not show my contempt in my voice—I asked him for a referral to a children's hospital in a neighboring state. He reluctantly agreed, but again said that he didn't know how the mother would be able to get the daughter to the appointment. I told him that I would take them.

This story has a happy ending. I did get the child and her mother to the hospital. She had the required test which showed that she did have epilepsy (a seizure disorder), was placed on medication and, as far as I know, is doing well today.

Our job as certified school nurses is to be advocates for the children in our care. When neither the child nor their parents are able to speak up, we need to do it for them.

To contact Caroline Champion, send an email to cchamp@stclair.k12.il.us.

A Life-Saving Assessment

By Judith Gerling, BSN

This is a story validating why we need to keep skilled nurses in our schools. Critical thinking is our forté and this ability comes only from a quality nursing education.

My story begins relatively innocently on a Monday in October in the health room of a large middle school. I was working with my aide giving routine vision and hearing screenings to our seventh grade students. My aide was giving a brief demonstration to a group of five students regarding what was expected of them during the screenings and, in a matter of seconds, a student named Alex fell into a sound sleep accompanied by loud snoring. After I awakened him and got his attention, I noticed dark circles under his eyes and wondered if he was experiencing sleep deprivation.

My suspicions were confirmed the next day. Alex was referred to me because of extreme lethargy in the classroom. He was demonstrating signs and symptoms of sleep apnea, a disorder characterized by periods of an absence of attempts to breathe. I had him lay down in my office and within seconds he fell asleep and was snoring loudly. In a short time, he began to exhibit involuntary movements of the extremities. This was followed by complete silence; in fact, he was so quiet that I wasn't sure if he was still breathing. But wait....he started snoring loudly again and made lots of flailing movements with his arms and legs. Then again, a period of absolute silence—was he still breathing? This sequence of behavior continued until I woke him up.

I immediately notified his mother and relayed my concerns of a possible sleep disorder. I encouraged her to seek a physician and suggested that a sleep study be administered as soon as possible. She had never witnessed these signs and symptoms before and asked me to be an advocate and write down my findings for the doctor. She was concerned that since Alex was autistic, his symptoms might be attributed to his autism and not be treated. Alex was often irritable and agitated, missed a lot of school and had difficulty remaining focused in the classroom. He was also often sick and a bed-wetter; the list goes on-and-on.

Several weeks later a sleep study was done and, indeed, my assessment turned out to be a life-saving one. During a 50 minute sleep study, Alex experienced 255 periods of apnea with no evidence of REM sleep! He was given a diagnosis of obstructive sleep apnea which had led to a central sleep apnea; a form of sleep apnea resulting from a decreased respiratory center output.

The doctor, fearing Alex would go into acute pulmonary failure, ordered a CPAP machine to maintain continuous positive airway pressure during sleep. Several weeks later, Alex had a T&A to relieve the obstruction. And guess what? His mother reports Alex is a different kid!

"You saved his life," she told me. He became more focused in school, improved his grades, had fewer absences, was less irritable and there was no more bed-wetting.

There is more to this story. Alex's mom stated that because of my accurate assessment and action, she was able to recognize similar symptoms in her younger son and seek medical advice much sooner. Fortunately, his sleep apnea was diagnosed at a much earlier age and he also underwent a T&A to correct his obstruction.

I thought to myself, *nurses really do make a difference in our schools—one skilled assessment at a time.*

To contact Judith Gerling, send an email to iwgerlin@smsd.org.

Tenacity

The author's name has been omitted to ensure that the identities of the individuals in this story remain confidential.

I remember well the first time I saw A.J. It was kindergarten round-up day and he was hard to miss. He had flawless skin the color of coffee and cream, curly brown hair and glasses as thick as Coke bottles. He was also all over the place and couldn't seem to follow directions. His mother seemed resigned as she told me, "He's nothing like his sister Amber. He's a handful."

Now I heard that many times, but busy little pre-school students often settle into kindergarten without any problems, so I wasn't concerned. I was curious about the glasses though, and asked A.J.'s mother if he needed accommodations for visual concerns. "No," she said. "He sees the eye doctors at the medical center every year and they say he can see fine with his glasses."

A.J. had an older sister at our school and a younger brother at home. His parents worked at minimum wage jobs, loved their children dearly and would do anything to help them succeed. A.J.'s healthcare was covered through an HMO, which accessed physicians at a major university teaching hospital.

School started in the fall and it was not long before the kindergarten teacher was at my door. "Could you come and observe A.J.?" she asked with a worried frown on her face. "I don't think he can see. He always wants to sit on my lap when I read. And it bothers the other children that he touches them a lot."

I went to the classroom and observed. I promptly screened A.J.'s vision and he failed. I called his mom who was most cooperative. Just three months before the start of school she took A.J. to the eye clinic but said she was willing to go again if I thought there was a problem. They went to the eye doctor and a referral form came back stating that A.J. could see within normal limits. A behavioral plan was put in place and accommodations were made.

First grade was a repeat of kindergarten. A.J. put his head down on his paper to try to write, would not follow directions, and played or was disruptive during group activities. He failed his vision screening once again and his mother marched back to the eye clinic. Again they returned with a referral form stating that his vision was fine as long as he wore his glasses. Attempts to improve his behavior were once again ineffective and after I met with his parents numerous times, a decision was made to have A.J. evaluated at the local mental health center. They thought perhaps he had ADHD. The diagnosis came back as childhood depression and he was put on medication.

The end of first grade and the beginning of second grade were a fog. A.J. was a zombie. His academic progress was poor—he just was not learning. In the classroom, he held his head cocked to the side, he put his face almost on his paper to write, and paid no attention to the overhead. He again failed the vision screening that I gave him but referral papers to the physician were returned once again stating his vision was within normal limits. The parents related that A.J. was a good basketball player and could play Nintendo at home so they didn't think his problem was vision. When I asked where he sat to play Nintendo, his mother replied that he would sit right in front of the TV about four inches away from the screen. She thought he did this just to make his brother and sister mad.

No course of action or attempted accommodations were working to improve A.J.'s learning development. We were puzzled. We even gave him an educational evaluation which indicated that he had normal intelligence. In desperation, I asked his parents for a release of medical information so we could see if there was documentation from any of his eye exams that would give us an indication of needed accommodations. A.J.'s parents were willing to try anything.

The medical release was sent to the eye clinic and the records arrived. The most recent report read: *20/40, 20/40???? Uncooperative.*

I looked back to the previous year's results which read: *20/40, 20/40?? Difficult to test*. Each year the results were marked with question marks and comments indicating testing concerns. A.J.'s mother told me that they often waited over five hours at the eye clinic before A.J. was tested. She noted that these long waits made A.J. tired and irritable.

I was more convinced than ever that a visual problem existed. With the parent's permission I called the eye clinic and was referred to a liaison nurse. I identified myself and requested information about the results of A.J.'s last vision exam. She pulled the records and, after a period of silence, said that she would get the physician who tested A.J. and asked me to hold.

The physician came on the line and in a brusque tone informed me that A.J. was uncooperative and hard to screen, but that his activities indicated that he could see. He went on to say that he did not have time to discuss such nonsense with a school nurse and *hung up!*

As I sat there pondering my next move the phone rang—it was the liaison nurse. She said she could have A.J. in to see the head of the department and asked if I would make sure he got to the appointment. I assured her that A.J. would come to the clinic on time and called his mother. She made quick arrangements to get off work to take A.J. to the appointment.

Late the next afternoon, A.J.'s mother called and said that he would be late to school the next day. A.J.'s exam had just ended and their new doctor said that he had a significant problem with his retinas and needed to see a retinal specialist the next morning. She also commented that they had a great appointment, didn't have to wait to be seen, and the doctor diligently worked with A.J.

The appointment with the retinal specialist resulted in a big shock for everyone. A.J.'s mother arrived at school and sat heavily in the only chair in my office. I closed the door.

"A.J. is blind", she said. "He has just a few pinpoints of vision on the outer perimeters of his eyes. The specialist said that his retina was scarred—probably from some type of virus when he was two or three years old. It can't be corrected. He says we need to teach A.J. Braille." She burst into tears and asked, "How could he play basketball and Nintendo without vision?"

It wasn't long before she pulled herself together; she wanted to do everything possible to help A.J. succeed. We contacted the district vision specialist to quickly put accommodations into place to maximize what vision A.J. had. He also began learning Braille with the vision specialist after school.

While a majority of our healthcare providers are wonderful, parents are sometimes hesitant to ask questions or request information because they feel inadequate in their relationship with professional staff. Those parents sometimes need help advocating for their children in the healthcare system. The school nurse is the person they often go to for help.

A characteristic that is most times left out when describing school nurses is tenacity. Yet, most school nurses can share time after time when tenacity was the characteristic needed to make certain that children's needs are fulfilled.

Email macgill@magill.com for information on how to contact the author of this story.

Running for Her Life

By Rose Magner, MSN, APRN, BC

I was working as a high school nurse in the small town where I lived when Haley entered the clinic one hot and humid afternoon in late August. She had changed into running shorts for her afternoon practice with the cross-country team. I noticed how thin Haley had become over the summer. Her cheeks were hollow, her collarbones protruded through her tee shirt and her eyes were sunken and surrounded by dark shadows. Always one of the fastest runners in our county, Haley informed me her goal was to become first in state in her division. She told me proudly that she was running several miles every day and working out with weights. I was so stunned by her appearance that I could only mutter "good luck" as she ran down the hall for practice.

I began to consider the implications of Haley's appearance. It was obvious her body was not receiving enough calories to meet her needs. What method was Haley using to achieve this weight loss? Dieting, exercise, starvation, and vomiting were all methods used by teens in our community. I knew I needed to involve myself quickly with Haley in order to make an initial assessment, and decided to start informally by inviting team members in for Gator-Aide before they left school for their afternoon runs.

I had learned about eating disorders from textbooks and lectures, but most of my knowledge came from my work with adolescents. I knew the signs and symptoms: an intense fear of fat, eating only small portions or not eating at all, exercising excessively, and weight loss, to name a few.

A pattern began to emerge over the next few days. Several students stopped in for drinks, including Haley. Haley always weighed herself first on the scale and become quite agitated if the number she desired did not materialize. She never drank Gator-Aide; a few sips of water were all she wanted. Her interactions with other members of the team became almost negligible, she rarely spoke to her peers and when she did it was in a very "bossy" or superior manner. This was very unlike the Haley I knew from previous years who had always been a team player, encouraging everybody to do his or her best. I realized intervention was required and privately asked Haley to meet with me the next day.

Haley was a bit leery of my intentions as she came to the clinic the next afternoon. I commented in my most non-judgmental fashion that I couldn't help but notice how much weight she had lost since the last school year. Would she share what she was doing to achieve these results? Haley's face brightened! Food, exercise, and weight loss were topics that she enjoyed discussing! Haley's general knowledge of nutrition, vitamins and minerals was impressive for a seventeen-year-old girl. She was always a dedicated student and a high achiever. She was simultaneously enrolled in challenging high school and college classes, visiting universities and filling out applications while training vigorously.

Haley was an only child of a prominent couple in our community. Her father was a well-known businessman active in several community boards and her mother had elevated volunteering to a fine art. Both had high expectations for their only child. Haley's father had attended a university on a running scholarship and it was his fondest dream that Haley follow in his footsteps. He was always generous with advice before and after every race. Haley's mother was a silent observer.

Over the next few weeks, Haley revealed that she wanted to attend a small religious college without a track program, but her father refused to allow it. He admonished her to work hard in order to receive either an academic or track scholarship, or both. He informed Haley that he expected her to attend the same university that he attended.

During this time Haley's weight continued to drop. Telltale signs, including reading in the library during lunch, bad breath, swelling around her jaw and mouth, skin breakouts, and frequent trips to the bathroom were all apparent. She was now running for an hour before school as well as with the team, fueled almost completely by caffeine. I was concerned that Haley might collapse during a run.

I called a friend who is a therapist to discuss the situation "in general." She recommended that I ask her running coach to become involved. She thought a pact would be a great idea. Haley would not be allowed to run with the team if her weight, blood pressure and pulse did not meet certain parameters. It was also time to get her parents actively involved.

When I brought these suggestions to Haley, she began to cry. She did not want her parents involved in any way. I discussed the importance of enlisting their support and informed her I was increasingly concerned about her health and safety. I explained the necessity of informing her parents and stated that I would if she had not by the end of the week. We role-played the discussion to help Haley become comfortable, and she thought she could tell them herself.

The decision to speak to Haley's parents if she could not caused me some anxiety. I knew it would destroy the tenuous relationship we had established. However, it was essential to bring Haley's behavior under control quickly as eating disorders are potentially fatal. Haley clearly needed more help than I was able to provide.

Unfortunately, Haley was losing her ability to relate to both her parents and her peers. She was becoming socially isolated and not able to maintain or establish a connectedness with others. She was not able to speak to her parents, and so I invited Haley's parents to attend a meeting with their daughter, her running coach, the two school counselors, and myself. Haley refused to attend the meeting at the last minute and her parents denied that they saw anything wrong with her appearance. They asserted she was simply training hard and probably not getting enough sleep. They did not understand why she would be penalized by not being allowed to run with the team. They would ensure that she went to bed earlier.

After her parents left, the counselors, coach and I sat in stunned disbelief. Where could we go from here? Haley's appearance continued to degenerate quickly. Her once shiny, thick auburn hair was becoming lifeless and dull and was falling out in clumps. She began wearing a baseball hat to cover the bald spots. Her eyes became listless, her smile rare, her bones jut through her clothes like knives.

One afternoon a short time later I was frantically summoned to a classroom over the intercom system. A student had collapsed, fallen, and hit her head. It was not surprising to discover the frail form of Haley crumpled in the pool of blood on the classroom floor. I was unable to wake her, but a faint pulse was palpable. An ambulance was sent immediately and we prayed this would serve as a wake-up call to her parents.

Haley was admitted to the hospital for severe dehydration, electrolyte imbalance and malnutrition. Her mother called the next day in tears, asking for help. I immediately referred her to a therapist who had extensive experience with adolescents and eating disorders. The family was seen in the hospital and intensive therapy began. My hope was that Haley could now begin the healing process.

It took almost two months before Haley would speak to me. She felt I had betrayed her. The therapist knew all her secrets and Haley could not involve her in her deceptions. Over time, however, Haley displayed some signs of recovery and forgiveness. She was seen in the cafeteria eating a cookie! Her cheekbones did not look quite so hollow. Her clothes did not seem to hang quite as much. Unexpectedly, she showed up timidly at the clinic door one afternoon, gave me a hug with tears glistening in her eyes, and whispered, "Thanks for everything you did for me."

Haley's improvement was based on a collaborative effort of many school and health care personnel. The response of her family, her therapist, and her eventual willingness to accept the help offered were all essential elements in her recovery. Despite the fact that my initial intervention seemed to serve no purpose at all, Haley's mother sent a simple note to the principal and school board. She wrote, "Thank you for having the foresight to hire a school nurse. She helped save my daughter's life."

The Clinic

By Judith Dorward, RN, MSN

We have a beautiful new school that cost $57 million and is the most expensive high school ever built in the state. Our superintendent, quoted in the newspaper, said, "People think I ought to be apologizing for it, but I'm not about to. Enlightened people build fine schools for their citizens and don't begrudge it."

The faculty, who spent many years in college so they can teach here, thinks the campus looks like a college. Some of the children, who have never known anyone who attended college but have spent many Sunday afternoons visiting relatives in prison, think the school looks like a prison.

Administration proudly brings visitors on tours of the new campus. "This is the nurse's office," they are told as they tour my suite. Visitors are impressed. They are never told that the offices are empty four days a week. The visitors never ask. The students, however, ask, "Where were you when I needed help?" Many of the students at this expensive new campus are so poor they cannot afford eyeglasses, dentist visits or trips to the doctor when they are sick.

Once a month we have a clinic at this new school. It doesn't cost the district a penny and nobody from the central office has ever been there to see it. Children whose parents work but do not have insurance benefits can use the clinic. Children whose parents have lost their jobs but do not qualify for state-funded medical assistance can use the clinic. Kids who are over eighteen and are living on their own while attending school can use the clinic. Children of illegal immigrants who have no source of medical care can use the clinic.

Read about a few of the students seen.

Tracy came to the nurse's office because she had a plantar wart. Both of her parents worked at minimum wage jobs and did not have insurance or qualify for state assistance cards. After rent, food and shoes for their three children they have nothing left for medical care. Tracy was having a terrible time coming to school because of the painful wart which made walking a struggle. I told her about the clinic and she immediately wanted to know if her sister could also come. "Beth needs glasses, real bad," she said. Tracy's mother was relieved to be able to bring her children to the clinic, and said, "You don't know what it's like to see your children needing something and not being able to help them."

Another student was sent to the nurse's office by her teacher because of an infected finger. It was swollen and draining green pus, causing her pain and keeping her from having a decent night's sleep. Her mother worked but did not have insurance. The student was seen in the clinic and had a complete check-up. We discovered that she had a hemoglobin level of 5.4. She received a chit to pay for a visit to the emergency room for a repeat blood test and was prescribed iron. A month later, her hemoglobin had not improved and the clinic provided her with a referral to a specialty clinic. We suspected that she had an inherited blood disorder.

Children who have no other access to care come to the clinic for glasses, dental care, referrals for counseling and tests for TB and other communicable diseases. All care is free and does not cost the school district anything. After treatment, children do better in school because they can sleep free of pain and debilitating conditions that sap their energy and dull their minds.

Public officials need to realize that the 1950's are over. Donna Reed is not waiting at home with cookies and milk. She is divorced and working while trying to go to school so that someday she can get a job with benefits. Her kids have very real needs that can be addressed by caring and imaginative people who are at the school often enough to be available to children. Needs that cannot be satisfied by expensive bricks.

The Right to Question

By Kristine Hallberg, RN, BSN

Don't ever let someone tell you that school nursing is a retirement job. I was almost convinced of this until I realized that my job was actually what *I made it to be*. Since I found I had the autonomy to either do "what I had to" or what I thought needed to be done, I changed my title to reflect that. I am now the Health Services Director. I not only see and coordinate care for a portion of my 1,200 K-12 students every day, I also coordinate our Employee Wellness Program with representatives from six other schools within our employee insurance trust. It has been a very busy yet rewarding year.

I set myself up to feel good about what I do. I try to make a positive change with the actions that I take. Whether it is a student in the first grade, the tenth grade, a first year teacher, or the teacher in his or her last year before retirement, they all deserve the same. They all deserve my best.

I wish I was reciting one of those stories that makes you chuckle for days, but this story is about the need for standing up for what is right and that old-fashioned gut feeling. This story is about having courage to face confrontation and quite possibly criticism in our actions. My motto is as follows: *If I can justify my actions for the right reasons, they are worth the action.*

There is a saying that a little knowledge can hurt you. It seems like everyone becomes a medical professional in one area or another when they've been given a little knowledge. Parents working for physicians are often the biggest culprits. Using family members in the healthcare field to avoid physician visits and costs are an even bigger offender.

I had a student in kindergarten suffer an asthma attack early in the fall during gym class. He was so accustomed to tolerating this physical occurrence that he refused to stop his activity to ease his symptoms, causing the teacher to have to physically bring him to my office. By the time he arrived he was in status asthmaticus. He was not yet cyanotic, but sternal retractions were obvious to the teacher, who knew that wasn't normal. The child's parents didn't provide any documentation indicating a history of asthma so I used an emergency protocol for administering Maxair inhaler with subsequent parent and 911 notification. While the ambulance facility is close to our school, sometimes minutes are too long.

When the parent arrived she verbally relayed her child's history of asthma. Needless to say, there had been no attempts at controlling his asthma except treating episodic occurrences. I informed the parent that the student needed to be seen by a physician as soon as possible. His respiratory status was improving, but wheezing remained throughout his lung fields following the repeated inhalations he was allowed (may repeat q20 min. X 2).

My little guy did go to the doctor—the office that is. Who he saw and was treated by is still a mystery. He returned with a rotahaler of a steroid that is used for maintenance treatment of asthma and a physician's order that bore the "stamped" signature of a physician ordering me to administer in the case of an acute attack. I confirmed the maintenance designation of this medication by Physicians Desk Reference and two pharmacies (I often consult the local pharmacy due to their vast knowledge of the newest treatments/drugs being marketed and solicited to physicians). Not surprisingly, the child experienced another attack that day while at recess. I attempted to contact the physician's office earlier to confirm the order, but was told to call back the next day to speak to the patient's family relative who had written the order. The office inferred that the physician that had supposedly written the treatment order did not see him. I again treated him with a Maxair Inhaler per emergency protocol. I contacted the parent and gave an update on the child's condition and my reluctance to use the medication brought to me. She returned to pick up her son and answer my more detailed questions regarding what treatment her son was receiving at home. I urged her to consult with the *physician* this time and stressed the severity of her son's asthma which could be much better controlled. The child had evidently tolerated his asthma this way for quite some time. He thought his severe episodes and difficulty breathing were acceptable.

By this time, I was very uncomfortable with the treatment this child was apparently receiving. His asthma was severely limiting his activities. Gym class and outside recess were triggering acute attacks. His prescribed medication did not seem appropriate nor did the medication order appear to be authentic. Doubting that I would ever get through to the physician for a verbal conversation, I immediately wrote him with a copy of his order and stated specifics about the child's last two witnessed episodes at school. I received a reply, but not from the physician. The nurse practitioner in the office assured me she had been to a conference and that the rotohaler medication was a "new" and acceptable means of treatment for acute attacks. Meanwhile, the student's relative in the office became livid that I had written the physician and questioned the order. She had a lot to say, but I'm not sure she understood my position. If the child's initial visit and subsequent medication order were legitimate then all I was requesting was confirmation. I would not follow an order blindly that I was uncomfortable with. It was imperative that the physician confirm his order.

I still received no communication from the physician after a good deal of time had passed. The child returned to school with a Maxair Inhaler following his second episode. He used it daily, continued to wheeze a majority of the time, and returned to school with an Albuterol Inhaler due to his Maxair Inhaler being depleted. That order did bear the Physician's handwritten signature.

It is not wrong to question. We as nurses need to always justify our actions. We strive for responsibility and professionalism in our students, our peers and ourselves. I have a license that I put on the line everyday. The bottom line is always "what's best for the child."

My experience has shown me that asthma inhalers are the most widely abused prescription medications. Doctors tend to prescribe them as a means of pacifying parents when symptoms give rise to an illness with respiratory involvement, but not a true diagnosis of asthma. No parent likes to hear that an illness "just needs to run its course." Students then use these inhalers during periods of physical exertion when they become winded. They use them for increased attention while breath sounds and peak flow readings remain normal. No medical condition requiring treatment with a bronchodilator exists. Parents excuse students from gym classes due to asthma much too frequently. A properly treated individual with a true diagnosis of asthma has few limitations, if any, and regular exercise should be an important part of his or her routine for asthma control. As our physical education classes have grown increasingly more strenuous with increased running time and true physical exercise, so have our excuses for non-participation in the class. Is it truly surprising that our nation has an obesity problem of epidemic proportions? Asthma certainly should not be an excuse for limiting physical activity in a PE class. Chronic asthma students almost always exhibit excellent asthma control when they are on a daily regimen of medications and use an inhaler approximately 20-30 minutes prior to exercise.

School nurses should not let their knowledge and experience go untapped. We should use it wisely and often. A student's best interest is always at stake.

To contact Kristine Hallberg, send an email to khallberg@netnitco.net.

More Than Meets the Eye

By Anne M. Biddle, RN, BSN

The winter of 2003 was one that will not soon be forgotten on the East Coast, as we were bombarded with snowstorm upon snowstorm. Between storms, we were able to squeeze in a few days of school. On one of these days, a most astute teacher became aware that something very odd was going on.

One of her star students had been "blanking out" and staring into space during class. She told me that his eyes became glazed, fixed and seemed non-responsive for seconds at a time.

The student assured his teacher that he was fine and also made a point of saying that he did not have ADD. Still, something did not seem quite right—so much so that she came to me, the school nurse, with her concerns.

As we thought about it, we both remembered a very impressive in-service on epilepsy we had the fortune of attending when our school opened up the year before. We remarked on how amazing it was to think those brief "stares into space" can actually be petit mal seizures; a sign of something far more *serious* than *annoying* going on. It was because of that in-service, in conjunction with one sharp teacher, that a life was likely saved.

Just to be on the safe side, I called the student's mother to relay the teacher's observations in class. I also mentioned that her son had frequent headaches as well that, alone, were no cause for alarm, but could be very important in conjunction with his "blanking out" episodes. The mother also mentioned (and denied) ADD as a possible cause, stating, "we pretty much ruled that out." This struck me as a common reaction to new and/or possible diagnoses.

A day went by, we endured another storm and multiple snow days led straight into the weekend. Finally back to school on Monday, our student in concern seemed completely exhausted by the end of the day. By the time his bus arrived to drop him off at his stop, he could barely walk into his house. "My legs feel like two tons," he told his Mom.

Had he overdone it in the snow? Stayed up too late over the weekend? Just out of shape?

Luckily, his quick thinking mom remembered his teacher's comments and my call, and contacted a pediatrician immediately upon seeing her exhausted son. The boy was ordered to go straight to the local ER for evaluation.

They were there within the hour, and not a moment too soon. The paralysis was ascending and close to reaching his waist. By the time he was diagnosed, his life was in jeopardy.

"Guillian-Barre Syndrome" came off the tongue of the doctor. This ascending paralysis was the classic symptom, and all other clues leading up to that day began to make sense. Had they waited to be checked out, the paralysis would have reached the boy's lungs, and yes, this odd disease had been fatal before. It attacks randomly as a virus and a favorable prognosis depends largely on early intervention. Timely recognition of his symptoms and quick action allowed the child to make a full recovery after going through physical therapy and strength training.

I am thankful for observant, caring teachers every day. In this case, a teacher's gut instinct very likely helped save a student's life. As Helen Keller said, "alone we can do so little, together we can do so much."

To contact Anne Biddle, send an email to annebiddle@comcast.net.

Building Bridges Between Health and Education

By Deborah A. Greenawald, RN, MSN

Rene was just a ninth grade student when I first met her. In the rural school district in southeastern Pennsylvania where I work, she was a fairly typical teenager in general good health and focused on all things adolescent—peer relationships, looking good and fitting in. Although her family history had been tumultuous, she was now living in a large residential children's home where the support of a multi-disciplinary team of highly qualified and caring people was continuously available to her. She was an outstanding basketball player, academically average and the type of student who didn't want to take time out of her social or class schedule to seek out the school nurse. Among a population of over 800 students, Rene easily melted into the larger picture until, during her sophomore year, she began coming to my office with steadily increasing complaints of shortness of breath, chest discomfort and other vague symptoms.

For many young people, a school nurse is the first person to detect a potential medical problem. Based on her assessment, referral, follow-up and continuing care during the school day as indicated, a school nurse may, in many ways, have a significant impact on patient outcomes. For Rene, a phone call to the resident nurse at her home initiated an evaluation by a family physician and she was subsequently treated for an asthmatic condition. I would occasionally see her for complaints of fatigue, dizziness and joint pain, all of which would be noted in her school health record and reported to the resident nurse where she lived. The student's complex social life also frequently caused increased stress, which either exacerbated her medical condition or mimicked it, making it difficult to decipher between real and perceived medical problems. When, however, her symptoms persisted and worsened over the course of a year, a more thorough medical evaluation began.

Rene was still reluctant to come to my office and was often angry when her symptoms became so apparent that the teacher sent her to see me. Nevertheless, it fell to this nurse, the only RN in the school building, to be her in-school advocate and communicate the medical problems she was experiencing, as I understood them, to her teachers. As time went on, Rene and I began building a bridge of understanding and mutual respect. I tried to appreciate her anxiety related to her condition and she tried to appreciate my responsibility to her and the importance of reporting any problems she experienced during school.

Rene was eventually diagnosed with Primary Pulmonary Hypertension (PH), an extremely rare condition whose etiology is unknown. Thanks to the support of the community in which she was living, Rene was able to access the medical system and be treated by expert doctors at a large regional medical center and, when indicated, traveled to Philadelphia for a more specialized evaluation and treatment plan. From diagnosis until now, I have been her advocate and supporter at the school where she spends a large part of her time. Her condition has forced me to learn new medications and protocols and understand complex medical situations in which school nurses are seldom involved. Following her hospitalization earlier this year for the insertion of a Hickman Catheter for a continuous infusion of Flolan, it was my responsibility to inform the faculty and staff about the severity of her medical condition and the safety precautions related to her med-pump that needed to be implemented. I also reassured them of her competency for self-care and, especially, her need to be treated as normal as possible in school.

No one can tell what Rene's future holds. At present time, her medical team is optimistic that her current treatment will control her PH until a better option is discovered. However, there remains the chance that she will need a lung transplant. Now, as Rene quickly approaches graduation, she is making plans for a career in nursing, pursuing a dream not just for her own wellness but to be a part of the journey to wellness for others.

There are many who do not understand the multi-faceted role of the school nurse and, therefore, may minimize the importance of this particular professional in the school setting when staffing configurations and budget constraints are discussed. And yet, frequently, the school nurse is the only one prepared to understand and interpret a student's medical condition and the effect this may have on his or her educational program. The bridge which Rene has helped me build between her own health needs and her education runs parallel to the bridge between my own on-going education and the health needs of all school children and adolescents. This story, then, spans not just the experiences of a nurse working to improve the health outcomes of her adolescent population, but also highlights the journey of a very extraordinary student. The efforts of nurses, including me, have indeed made Rene's life better. In return, however, by compelling me to once again build a bridge between health and education, she has made my life better and is a continuing reminder of the importance of what I do in school and community health.

The Nurse as a Catalyst

By Patricia L. Collier, RN, BSN, MA

I serve as a school nurse in a program for moderately to severely developmentally delayed students. We have many classes on regular school sites in our area. We also have a school site which serves those students whose special needs keep them from the regular school site. I make daily visits to the classes of most of these special needs students. This keeps me current on their nursing needs and makes me available to the staff. Because I have close contact with all staff working with students, I am sometimes the moving force behind changes needed to improve a student's program.

Richard was a nine-year-old boy who had contracted meningitis at the age of four and suffered severe brain damage. He came to our school at the age of five with a diagnosis of cerebral palsy and seizure disorder. Richard was unable to walk, talk or use his hands. He had lost vision in the lower half of his visual field and was fed by gastrostomy tube.

For the first few years Richard was with us, his program was very functional. He wasn't able to respond but was introduced to a lot of information. One day, while visiting another classroom, the teacher began asking Richard to point to colors as she said them. He was able to identify all the colors and could also identify numbers. It was evident that he had been learning all along but was unable to express what he knew.

At age nine, Richard was ready. I spoke to a teacher who was very good at understanding non-verbal communication and helping students find a way to communicate. Richard began spending time in her classroom.

When classes were being arranged for the new school year, Richard was not placed in the class with the teacher I thought he needed. The teacher and I put our heads together and decided that the best thing to do would be to ask Richard where he wanted to be during his annual IEP meeting. He was able to tell the team what class he wanted (he was able to answer yes and no questions at that time). The team then changed his class to the one he wanted.

Richard is now thirteen years old and has been in his new class for three years. He is using his second augmentative communication device (he quickly outgrew his first one) and will need an upgrade soon. He is able to say almost everything he wants to say. His mother says she has to turn off his machine at church because he talks too much. He eats by mouth now and uses his gastrostomy tube only for liquids. He was evaluated on a motorized wheelchair but the lack of lower vision impaired his ability to drive alone. We will work on teaching him to move his head to increase his visual field and then try again. Next year Richard will be moved to a regular junior high school campus in a special day class while beginning to mainstream into regular education. Richard is very excited and has plans to finish school, get a job and live on his own.

Although I can't take credit for any of Richard's educational progress, I am happy that my involvement aided in getting him the right teacher at the right time.

To contact Patricia Collier, send an email to collier_pat@lacoe.edu.

Complete Care: Physical, Emotional and Educational

By Marcia Lozes, CPNP

A seven-year-old first grader started coming to the nurse's office in September every day with harsh coughing that made her unable to perform class work. The school nurse assessed him and contacted the mother for further information. He was receiving some medication at home for asthma and we were able to help the mother by administering medication during the day at school. We also provided a place for him to rest when needed and to eat meals in privacy when he had coughing fits that made him prone to have emesis. This was a very attractive, personable and bright boy who liked school and was popular with his teacher and classmates.

Improvement was minimal at best and the nurse encouraged the mother to keep him on his medications, get adequate rest, and to return to his physician. The mother had a new baby and became frustrated with her seven-year-old's physician visits with no improvement and his need to be sent home everyday. She began taking him to other clinics for other opinions. Since his regular doctor is part of a large HMO with subspecialists, we encouraged her to continue his management with his regular doctor. We made sure to call his physician to report how poorly he was responding to his medication, how severe his symptoms were and the large amount of school he was missing. We continued to send notes to his doctor regarding his condition and absences.

Nine months after the start of the school year the student was diagnosed with Cystic Fibrosis and referred to a specialty clinic. His mother felt very comfortable to call the nurse to express her grief and sadness about his diagnoses. She helped to give the mother and teacher more information and encouragement regarding his follow-up. The nurse, attendance counselor and collaborative group at the school formed a plan to initiate home schooling and a special classroom placement to facilitate "catching-up" on his education. The nurse followed through with the doctor to get the home schooling request initiated and made sure everyone had adequate information for prompt admission.

Although the child had not yet been seen by the cystic fibrosis clinic, a great deal of intervention had already occurred though the efforts of the school nurse to coordinate an adequate assessment, communicate with the mother, teacher, attendance counselor and doctor. She was supportive with the child's mother as she dealt with his new diagnosis. The nurse even initiated a project with many of the staff and children to write him letters and let him know how much they missed him. The nurse was a key coordinator in managing all the aspects of getting this child adequate care medically, emotionally and educationally.

II

Beyond the Job Description

"I was reminded of how many Band aids and icepacks school nurses give to children, not only to treat physical pain, but to soothe emotional pain from wounds we may never know unless we take the time to listen."

— Lorali Gray, RN, BSN

Sara's Story

By Jeanne R. Sievers, RN

It was the very first day at a new school for Sara and me. I was the new high school nurse and Sara was the new ninth grader from a small town. The size of this urban school and the large amount of students enrolled was a little overwhelming for both of us.

The first day started with several crises at once. The first visitor to my health office was a ninth grader. She had a history of grand mal seizures and was having a rather severe episode. She went into status epilepticus and an ambulance was called. Next, an assistant principal brought a male student to me who was very upset (his brother had attempted suicide) and slept in the dugout at the baseball field on campus all night. Another student was vomiting with a high fever. Then Sara and her mom walked into my office. This all happened at virtually the same time.

Sara was a beautiful young girl with long brown hair and beautiful brown eyes. In my office, she was in tears and clinging to her mother who was also in tears. Her mother was obviously in great emotional pain over her daughter's unhappiness. Sara seemed very young, very innocent and terrified to be at such a large and unfamiliar campus. Mother and daughter waited patiently as I triaged my patients. Finally, I was able to talk with them and assess their situation.

Sara's mother explained that she was recently divorced and had just moved to the city from a small town with a small school. Sara didn't want to leave her friends, her family and the comforts of her old home and school. The weekend before school started she was extremely depressed and tried to end her life with an overdose of pills. She ended up in the hospital that weekend.

When I looked at the desperation in the eyes of both Sara and her mom my heart was overwhelmed with compassion and concern. I explained that I would take care of Sara that first terrifying day. I told Sara it was my first day too, and we would work through it together. When Sara said she didn't have anyone to eat lunch with, I let her know that I didn't have anyone to eat with either. I suggested that she eat with me in my office and she reluctantly agreed. I assured her mother that Sara would be okay and sent her on her way home.

My nephew was also a freshman on campus and I knew a few of his friends. I asked that they befriend Sara and asked each of her teachers to be particularly sensitive to her situation.

Sara arrived in my office at noon and we had lunch together. I tried to make her feel emotionally safe with me. She was very quiet and withdrawn but seemed to be doing okay. I told her we would make it through today a period at a time and then we would take it a day at a time. I went on to encourage her and tried to be sympathetic to her situation. The second day of school we continued our regimen and she seemed just slightly better.

A day or two later, I was picking up my son at middle school when I heard a loud yell: "Hey, Mrs. Sievers!" I looked across the parking lot and there was Sara and her mom picking up her younger brother. She and her mom had big smiles on their faces! I waved enthusiastically and was fully aware that I had a smile on my face as well.

As the year continued, Sara improved both academically and socially. She became very involved and successful. She was my student aide, was a delightful young lady and blossomed into a beautiful woman both inside and out.

On the first school day of the following year, when Sara was a sophomore, she and her mother sent me a beautiful bouquet of flowers in appreciation of what I had done for Sara. They attached a card that read: "Please know that you will be in our thoughts and prayers today and many tomorrows—and also for all the new students like Sara was last year, full of fear and anxieties. I know the Lord will lead those to you who need your special touch. Thanks again for being there when Sara needed you. To look at her now, you would never imagine what she was like at this time last year. Love, Karen and Sara."

There is more to this story. Sara and I had our first day at this high school in the fall of 1990. On the first day of school for the past twelve years—every year since 1990—I receive a glorious bouquet of flowers from these special people expressing their gratitude for the compassion and concern I showed Sara. I am so busy on that crazy first day of school that I am amazingly surprised when the flowers and special note arrive. My tears of joy and humility remind me of the incredible difference we can make in just one child's life. At the start of each year, this family's generous and appreciative hearts take me back to my first day on the job as the new high school nurse. From the moment those flowers arrive I am energized and encouraged to take care of "my kids" in whatever capacity I can.

Some days, in a school of 2200 students, my job can be extremely challenging and my patience can run thin. But when I think back to that very first day of school in 1990, I smile and say to myself, *the next kid that walks into my office could be another Sara.*

I am so grateful for Sara because she taught me so much about being a school nurse. It isn't just about taking care of physical needs, immunization laws and screening kids for vision, hearing and scoliosis. School nursing is about listening and genuinely caring for a child. As for Sara, she is now happily married to a wonderful man and has two beautiful children. We continue to stay in touch.

Band Aids and Icepacks: Beyond the Physical Pain

By Lorali Gray, RN, BSN

I remember that September day well. As a school nurse, I reported to one of my rural elementary schools that housed six hundred students in preschool through sixth grade. My head was swimming with the day's activities as I tidied the two-bed health room, all the while knowing that every day in school nursing is different, bringing both challenges and rewards. However, I had no way of foreseeing the lesson I would be reminded of that day.

As I began to prioritize my list of activities, the morning flew by. I was constantly aware of the clock as I knew lunch and recess were imminent. The experience of a school health room milieu during lunchtime and recess is unique! This day brought 22 students needing medication, a dressing change, a daily page for a diabetic student, a nebulizer treatment, a staff blood pressure check and countless others with injuries and illness.

When the lunchtime rush hit I had two ill students sleeping and was buried in immunization data needing to be compiled for an upcoming audit. As I looked up from my desk I saw the secretary escorting a kindergartener to the health room. "She got hit in the nose with a soccer ball," she stated. Blood was running down the girl's face as she made a feeble attempt to pinch her nose. I helped her in and had her sit down in the only available spot, the end of the bed that was already occupied by one of my malingering "regulars." Hysteria broke out as the other children were awakened to the sight of blood, causing increased anxiety and wailing from a kindergartener. As I put on my gloves to assist her, a young boy quietly walked into the chaos of the health room, handed me a note and stood waiting for direction. After stabilizing the nosebleed and calming the hysteria I read his note: *Mike to health room for ice pack; hurt leg.*

Mike had been referred by a playground supervisor after being kicked in the leg while playing soccer. After an assessment of his injury, I determined he needed a Band aid and icepack so I had him join the others by sitting on the last chair in the corner. Mike was a courteous unassuming boy who did not complain about his injury. He instead sat quietly with his icepack watching life in the health room. Thirty minutes later I realized that many children had come and gone while Mike remained sitting quietly with the icepack. His injury did not appear that serious to me, but for some reason he felt he needed to go home. I respected his decision and decided to call his parents. I started my routine set of questions: Is anyone home that can pick you up? Do your parents work? Do they speak English?

His answer took me by surprise: "My mother is at home. My father died last month."

Suddenly the health room became still, children were quiet and time seemed to stop. My mind cleared of my impending immunization audit, the family arriving in half-an-hour for a preschool health assessment and the other children in the room. As I rolled my chair across the tiny room to focus my attention on his response, I wasn't sure how to proceed. My gut reaction told me to just listen, and as I did, it became clear that out of the chaos of an elementary school health room a grieving boy had opened a door of opportunity for both himself and for me as he shared from his heart his experience with death. I felt an immediate calming as I listened to his story. I did not have to speak or fumble to fill the silence. All I needed to do was listen, which was apparently what Mike came to the health room to have me do. Listening can so often get lost in the daily challenges of school nursing. However, at that school, at that moment, for that child it was not physical pain that needed to be treated with a Band aid and ice pack but emotional pain that needed to be treated with a listening ear.

Later as I reflected on the day, I was reminded of a valuable lesson. Not from a professional journal, colleague, or institution of higher learning, but from a child. I was reminded to embrace the calm in the midst of the chaos, see the child in the midst of the children and hear the heartfelt story of a grieving child in the midst of those who malinger. I was reminded that day of how many Band aids and icepacks school nurses give to children, not only to treat physical pain, but to sooth emotional pain from wounds we may never know unless we take time to listen.

To contact Lorali Gray, send an email to lorali@mtbaker.wednet.edu.

An Obstacle Overcome

By Kristy Rasdall, RN

One of the best memories I have of my years as a school nurse is of a little special needs student named Anna. This story doesn't involve taking her temperature, cleaning her scraped knee, or administering medication; it is about helping her overcome a potentially huge obstacle.

Anna came to our school as a kindergartener and was mainstreamed with the help of a paraeducator throughout her elementary school years. As she grew up, her mother became concerned about how she would talk to her about normal growth and development and the menstrual cycle. When Anna began fifth grade, I consulted her mother regarding how to go about this instruction. As a result of our discussion, I talked with Anna about what to expect. Twice that year, I showed her a video which was geared exclusively towards special needs girls. Each time I showed Anna the video, she would practice pad changes and disposal and would repeat—almost word for word—parts of the video back to me.

When Anna started sixth grade I again talked with her mother regarding growth and development instruction and showed Anna the video several times. That year, Anna actually began practicing being on her period. She would apply a sanitary pad to her underwear in the morning when she arrived, change it every four hours, and dispose of it properly. We repeated these practice sessions each month until the end of the year. When sixth grade came to an end, Anna had still not started menstruating. Nevertheless, I assured her mother repeatedly that, after watching her practice, I thought she would handle it absolutely fine.

Sure enough, the summer after sixth grade, I got a call from Anna's mother. She told me that Anna had started her first period about a week after school was out. Amazingly, when her mother discovered that she had started, she also found out that Anna had actually started four days earlier and had taken care of everything by herself—without even telling her mother.

I felt so happy for both of them. Anna had to have felt so successful and proud that she had started and was able to take care of herself without help. And her mother must have felt much more at ease knowing that her special needs daughter was able to take care of this monthly occurrence on her own. She now knew that in years ahead, when she may not always be available to offer help, Anna could handle it.

I feel as if this is one of my biggest success stories. The success story, however, really belongs to Anna.

Healing Spirit

By Elvira O. Gonzalez, RN, BSN, MA

"Hi, Mrs. Gonzales," Jason said as he limped into my office. "Hi Jason," I chided. "You back again?" I knew Jason fairly well throughout his high school career as he visited my office quite often. He came in with ailments ranging from headaches and skin rashes to bumps and bruises. I half-suspected that he simply needed a diversion from his classes. Jason was not the most academically driven type, but I found him endearing for his polite and pleasant manner. He was always eager to just sit and converse—perhaps he sought out that extra attention that most high school students crave. I laughed to myself thinking, *where better to receive tender loving care on demand but from a nurse's office?* "What happened to your ankle?" I asked.

"I sprained it playing basketball in Phys. Ed.," he said to his chagrin. Jason was on the school basketball team and though he was not the star player, his athletic ability was enough to keep him competitive.

"Oh, no. I guess you can't walk through commencement," I joked. "Here, take a seat and I'll bandage you up."

Jason limped to the chair and seemed a little preoccupied. Commencement exercises were just three days away, and from my experience working at schools, students usually became anxious around graduation time each year.

"So," I said trying to ease the strain creeping across Jason's face, "what college will you be attending after graduation?"

Jason looked up at me with surprise. "Mrs. Gonzales, I'm not going to be attending college. You know that I'm barely passing my classes now. I'm going to continue working at my minimum wage job...my dad said I should just keep trying to make some money so I can eventually support myself."

I looked Jason in the eyes and said, "Just because you're not doing well in high school doesn't mean you can't do well in college. Why don't you at least consider first attending the community college? They have two-year transfer programs to universities."

Jason looked down and watched me as I finished ace-wrapping his ankle. After a couple of minutes he asked, "Why do you think I'd be able to get into college? My parents don't even think college would be an option for me."

I sat down in the chair next to him. "Jason," I said with emphasis, "your life is just beginning after graduation. You need to discover your skills as a growing adult." I went on to explain that in life people do not have to live with any one set of circumstances. People have choices. This young man could either stay working at a minimum-wage job for years or choose to make something more of his life. Jason nodded his head and smiled politely. I could tell that he wanted to believe something more was possible than being stuck "barely getting by" for the rest of his life.

"When you get home this evening," I continued, "sit down in your room and think about what we talked about. Think about all that it has taken for you to just get through high school and play basketball. You had to work really hard maintaining your grade-point eligibility to stay on the team. You don't know what you're capable of until you try. Reflect on what you want in life and what you see yourself doing. Hopefully, some good decisions will be made." Jason left my office that afternoon without saying much more.

As I was boxing up the remaining items to close out the school year I heard a light knock at my door. It was Jason. "Hi, miss me already?" I said with a smile. "Are you ready for graduation tomorrow?"

Jason shyly nodded his head. "Mrs. Gonzales, I just wanted to thank you for taking time to talk to me the other day," he said. "I wanted to let you know that my sister is taking me to the community college to register for classes tomorrow." He then walked over and gave me a bear hug. "I'm glad I sprained my ankle ... otherwise I wouldn't have gotten to talk to you. You've really changed my thinking. I've got to make my own decisions now and take my own actions as to how my life should end up. Thanks for making me see that."

As we parted ways my heart swelled with pride. I was reminded that simple words were enough to impact life changes. Raising the bar and having higher expectations for our students is all that some of them need to push themselves and reach higher goals. When students come to visit the nurse's office they sometimes seek more than medical attention. Sometimes motivating students simply requires an understanding ear to listen and words of comfort or praise. I was reminded that as a school nurse I am not only here to help bandage wounds but also to help heal broken and wavering spirits.

To contact Elvira Gonzalez, send an email to cjoydunham1@aol.com.

Terri

By Nancie Rodriguez, RN, BSN, PHN

I first met Terri when I worked for the Office of Education in a major city. I was the school nurse for twelve pregnant and parenting teen programs and six community education centers. I was screening the students at a Middle School CEC for hearing and vision and it was quite difficult. Students enrolled at this school were there because they had no where else to go. They all had discipline problems, had been expelled from regular public schools and were trying to finish the school year. The teachers were not very cooperative in helping me set up and structure the screening so I could finish. Finally, I grabbed a girl and asked her to help by getting the kids from their classes. She seemed really happy to help and was very sweet. Her teacher later told me that she was expelled form her high school for selling ecstasy to middle school kids. One boy had taken it at school and had a full blown seizure.

A year later, I changed jobs and was working at the high school in the same city. One day, a school counselor brought a girl to the health office. In strict confidentiality, she told me that the girl had been complaining about difficulty urinating and pain. I did an assessment with the girl and she had symptoms of a UTI and possibly an STD. She refused a referral to a doctor stating that she did not have one. She went on to say that she couldn't go to a doctor with her mother because she didn't want her to find out that she was sexually active. She was also breaking the conditions of her enrollment by getting back together with her boyfriend.

I realized that this was Terri, the girl from the CEC that had helped me with the screenings. Since leaving the CEC, she had been given strict guidelines to stay away from her boyfriend and attend high school. I made an appointment for her at a free clinic located about ten miles from school. She had no way to get there, so I took her.

We waited about two hours for her to be seen and then another hour for her prescription to be filled. While we waited, we watched television talk shows and chatted. She remembered helping me at the CEC and felt comfortable sharing her problems. Her mother was from another country and very traditional. She spoke no English and had a younger boyfriend living in the home who she was trying to become pregnant with. She had Terri at 16. There was no father.

We went to lunch after making another appointment for Terri to have a Pap in anticipation of getting some form of birth control. At lunch, I told her that I had a daughter the same age and spoke of my concerns about young girls getting involved sexually. I talked to her about the way I parent my children and about my values regarding relationships, maturing, education and her future.

The following week, I took her to another appointment. Afterward, I took her to lunch again, we talked more about her situation and she asked about my relationship with my daughter. I encouraged her to confide in her own mother and to trust her mother to continue to love her.

After several months, she returned to my office and asked that I help one of her friends. She had been getting a Depo-Provera shot every three months and had several friends that wanted this as well. I showed them how to make an appointment at the free clinic and how to take the bus there. I also took them to a pregnancy prevention conference at St. Anne's, a maternity home. In addition, we started a teen issues support group which unfortunately came to an end when all of the girls participating were failing the fifth period class time we were using.

Terri continued to come to the health office periodically. She came for help in finding a new clinic when the one she used closed and when her friends thought they might be pregnant. She brought her boyfriend in one day when he was ill, and we referred him to our district health center.

Her grades began to rise and went from D's and F's to C's. One day, she came to the office crying because her counselor wanted her to take biology and algebra and she was terrified. We talked though her fear and she decided to go ahead and try the classes.

Later, her best friend got pregnant and all three of us sat there and cried before we told her mother. Terri continued to stay close to her friend and brought her to me weekly for advice, encouragement and even celebration after her first ultrasound picture.

Terri still comes to the health office to "hang out" about every two weeks. She is taking chemistry in the fall and her grades have climbed to the A and B range. She wants to become a nurse, perhaps working with adolescents, and hopes to attend college with the help of scholarships or loans. She also would very much like to meet my daughter and tell her how lucky she is.

To contact Nancie Rodriguez, send an email to rodriguez_n@sgusd.k12.ca.us.

A Very Special Christmas

By Darlene A. Wynn, MSN, PNP

I have been a school nurse for 20 years and have had countless experiences—from caring for students with medical disorders to disgruntled parents. However, the memory of one particular Christmas will remain with me forever.

It was the day before Christmas vacation and excitement could be felt in the air. Voices of middle school children were a bit louder than usual and other students were going from room to room singing Christmas carols. Bits of Christmas wrapping paper could be found on the hall floors after gift exchanges between friends. Everyone anxiously awaited the bell to go home early for the holiday.

Before the break could officially begin, I had to call a parent to follow up on an illness that a child had presented earlier in the week. I called the child's mother and in the process of the conversation, I wished her a happy holiday. She responded by telling me that it would not be a happy holiday for her family. She said that she had six children, a husband that did not have a job, and—with Christmas just two days away—there was no money available for gifts. I looked at the clock which read 1 p.m. The school dismissal was at 1:30 p.m. I replied by saying that her children would have a Christmas. I had no idea how I would accomplish this task but I was certain to make it happen.

I called the local television station to inquire regarding a commercial for Toys for Tots where toys were collected by the US Marine Corp. I was given an address where one could pick up donated toys; the donating site was in the city and not too far from where my husband worked.

I called my husband and asked him for help. He took the ages and genders of the children and hopped a bus to get to the distribution center before it closed. I grabbed a hat and began to take up a collection from the teachers, staff and administration.

At the end of the day, my husband came home with some toys but not one for every child. We took the money and added some of our own and went shopping. We ended up with several boxes of toys and food for the family.

That night my husband, myself and my children loaded up our car with the gifts. I will always remember what a cold crisp night it was. There were just a few snow flakes drifting from the sky. We drove up to the house and knocked on the door.

When the door opened it was a sight to behold. A curtain separating the stairway from the front room hung from a rod. The curtain was closed but through the center opening of the curtain there were six little heads, one on top of the other, peering at us. The children never moved but just watched. The mother said thank you and wished us a very Merry Christmas. I know it was the merriest I had ever had.

To contact Darlene Wynn, send an email to dwynn@westallegheny.k12.pa.us.

Shoes

By Deborah H. Turley, RN, BSN, NCSN

As a school nurse I sometimes get a little frustrated about the nature of the care I am asked to provide. I expect to deal with the never-ending stream of students with minor complaints and the acute and serious situations arising from asthma attacks, sickle cell crisis, diabetic hypoglycemic reactions and psychological problems. On a recent day when I had dealt with all of these in a four hour period, I was less than pleased when I received a nurse referral for a child whose feet hurt. The child was in pain because she put her shoes on the wrong feet, a detail I felt her teacher could have noticed and cured.

After I switched the shoes to their correct position and sent the child happily on her way, I was reminded of another recent shoe incident. One of my more challenging students with asthma had come in for her morning peak flow reading. I had prided myself on my active case management of this student. I educated her in doing peak flow readings to manage her asthma, helped her family to obtain financial assistance to secure medication, assisted in getting her a primary care provider, and had emergency appointments scheduled for her on several occasions when she did not respond to nebulized medication at school. On this particular day, however, I just small-talked and asked her about her spring break. Expecting a recitation of all the wonderful things children do on a break from school, I was surprised to hear her say, "Terrible."

"Why, what happened?" I asked.

"Well, I was sick all week. But what was really bad was that I didn't get to go to the Easter egg hunt at church because I didn't have any church shoes."

I thought of the three pairs of Easter shoes I had just purchased my daughters. One pair didn't fit as we had expected, size three being just a little too small.

"What size shoes do you wear, sweetheart?" I asked.

"Three," she replied. A quick look at the shoes she was wearing confirmed this to be true.

The next day she was thrilled when she received a gift from my youngest daughter, a pair of white, size three dress shoes. Her smile lit up my office.

When I got home that afternoon, my daughter asked me if I had given the little girl her shoes. When I told her that I had and that the little girl loved them, her smile was just as bright as the recipient's had been. Another of my daughters said, "Mom, look at all the shoes we got today!"

Sitting in my living room floor were two large sized garbage bags filled with shoes from a church friend with daughters older than mine. Inside were pairs and pairs of tennis shoes, sandals, school shoes, and a single pair of white dress shoes—size four—just the right size for my daughter.

What do shoes have to do with school nursing? While I am sure that this child appreciated all the times I have cared for her asthma exacerbations, I had never seen her smile quite like I did when she received the gift of shoes. Nor did the child with her shoes on the wrong feet care why they hurt as much as she cared that I could make her feel better. In a child's world it is often the little things that mean the most. I was reminded of one of Mother Teresa's sayings: "One can do no great things, only small things with great love."

To me, that is the essence of school nursing.

To contact Deborah Turley, send an email to debtimt@aol.com.

Reassurance

By Susan Reiss, RN, NCSN

An interesting thing happened on the third day of a new school year. Sometimes we just don't realize how important the little things we do or say mean to someone. On this day during mid-morning, a little girl came to my office and was very upset because of a loose tooth she had been trying to remove for two months. It was slightly bleeding and painful for the young girl. I cleaned her mouth, numbed it up and told her that "today would be the day" the tooth would come out.

An hour later, she was back and said her tooth hurt again. I told her it was too soon to numb it again but it was even looser than before and wouldn't be long before it came out. She seemed okay and went back to class.

I then went to lunch and, before long, the assistant principal interrupted me and said that a little girl was sobbing hysterically outside my office—something about a tooth (it's true that school nurses are unable to get a 15 minute, uninterrupted lunch). Sure enough I found the girl sobbing on my cot because, as she put it, her tooth was so loose that it kept hitting the tooth above it and she couldn't eat and hadn't eaten breakfast. Being a take-charge kind of person and also a real softie for crying little girls, I asked her to show me what she had for lunch. She pulled out a fluffer-nutter sandwich and I exclaimed that it was perfect! I showed her how to remove the crust and break off tiny bits and chew them on the other side of her mouth. Once she got the hang of it we explored the rest of her lunch. I told her the eight sandwich cookies would have to wait, but by the evening I was sure she would be able to eat them also. I talked her into going back to the lunchroom and she said she would be okay. I settled her in with some girls and at 1 p.m. she came back to my office and said her tooth was almost out. She was so proud that she not only ate the entire sandwich but was able to share her friend's French fries as well. She wanted to try to remove the tooth herself; I agreed and gave her a gauze pad.

One minute later she ran out in front of me, so proud of her pulled tooth and sticking her tongue through the hole where it used to be. I then asked if the tooth fairy came to her house and she said, with tears in her eyes, "My mom knows about the tooth fairy, but I don't know if my dad does, you see, we have to live with my dad now."

We explored ways to let her dad know what happened and about tooth fairy traditions. She left my office beaming and said it was the best day ever! I will never forget how important empowering children and giving them a moment of caring and comfort can be. It goes a long way to offer reassurance in a sometimes difficult world.

If you would like to contact Susan Reiss, send an email to sreiss@sanborn.k12.nh.us.

A Family in Need

By Peggy Six, RN

It was brought to the attention of the school team that one of our sixth grade students had numerous absences and had not been attending school for several consecutive days. To address the issue, one of our administrators held a conference call with the student's mother. I was included on the call along with the school guidance counselor. She told us that she was a single mother who recently had surgery, needed to wear a neck brace and was using a walker to ambulate. In addition to her sixth grade son, she also had a four-year-old and a two-year-old daughter. She was keeping her son home to care for his sisters.

I was asked to intercede to try and find help so the sixth grader could return to school. I called social services and explained the situation. Social services were willing to attempt to provide aid, but were unable to contact the family via telephone. I made a home visit only to find that the family's phone services had been turned off and they were in danger of being evicted.

I contacted social services again and, working in coordination, we were able to provide the family with food, emergency stipends for rent and money for an aide to come to the home and provide care. After having taken these steps, the often-absent student was able to return to school.

The Best Christmas Ever

By Connie Racine, RN

I have been a school nurse for several years and have had many memorable moments, but the one that sticks out in my mind was the year that our school and community came together to make one family's Christmas their best ever. A single mother with five children lived in our town—the oldest was 11 and the youngest was in pre-school. The mother supported her family by working as a waitress at a local restaurant and received no other financial support. She was a proud person.

The home they rented was poorly insulated and required more for heating than the mother could financially afford. There would be no Christmas for this family. How could we, the school, help this mother with the approaching Christmas season?

I wrote a letter as Santa Claus to the K-12 school staff. The letter contained information about the family without using a last name. It included some humor; mentioning staff that was "naughty and nice," Santa's age and the fact that he needed help. If our staff wanted to be guaranteed a surprise from Santa that year, I wrote, he needed them to think of the less fortunate and grant him, Santa, a wish. Santa wished to make Christmas for this family of six "the best ever."

I expected a response from the elementary and middle school staff but the overall community response was overwhelming. Word spread to our rural community that usually stayed to themselves; they more or less felt the school had "enough" and that teachers were overpaid. I could not in my wildest dreams have imagined the overwhelming support that came forth.

We set aside space for gifts in the teachers' room, and the collection steadily grew. Local stores donated coupons for merchandise to include food, clothing, film processing and fuel. People donated money to purchase a Christmas tree with decorations, a complete Christmas dinner with all the fixings, gift certificates and enormous food donations. Teachers and other volunteers came together to wrap gifts with donated wrapping paper and bows. I noticed during this period of time that the staff complained less, smiled more, laughed more, were excited about the holidays, and thought less about their own needs.

Days before Christmas, I stood in the gift room in amazement at all the brightly wrapped gifts, boxes of food, and a Christmas tree with boxed decorations. My last concern was finding a way to transport these many carloads of gifts to the family's home.

A local fireman who dressed each year as Santa called me and said he would love to dress as Santa and have someone drive him to the family's home in a fire truck with all the gifts. I called the mother and told her that I had some things to deliver to her home to help with Christmas, and asked her to be sure that her kids were out of the house for a little while.

The Saturday before Christmas, my youngest son and I met "Santa" and his driver at the school. We loaded my car and the fire truck with boxes of gifts and food. With Santa holding on to the back of the fire truck, his driver drove him to the home of the family and I followed behind with my son. As we drove up the driveway, the truck's siren rang out and a joyous "HO, HO, HO" was blasted through the loud speaker.

There are two things that I will always remember about that day. The look on the mother's face that no words could express and a comment from my son: "Thanks, Mom." My children had never been without food and for my son to experience first hand the emotion this mother of five exhibited made him appreciate what he had and realize what others go without. The family showed us their appreciation with a large poster of pictures of Christmas morning with words of thanks to Santa from each of them.

School nursing in my community isn't always about medical help. It's the spirit of offering our service beyond what we were trained to do. It's always about the kids.

To contact Connie Racine, send an email to cracine@dhhs.state.nh.us.

III

Finding Inspiration

"Sometimes it takes a child to show us
the best in ourselves."

—Kathy Borniger, RN

Facing Our Greatest Fear

By Jeannie Bower Edwards, RN

I feel that a school nurse has an extraordinary amount of responsibility to students and staff. In addition to being the only qualified medical expert in the school, the school nurse is often the first and only capable expert in the event of an emergency. I take my responsibilities seriously, my skills are competent and I teach CPR to keep these skills sharp. I do all that I physically can and leave the rest to the Lord. Each and every morning I pray for the health and safety of my staff and students and the wisdom and power to do my best. My greatest fear has always been that a child would be seriously or fatally injured and that I would fail in my attempt to rescue him or her. I knew that I would be devastated if I ever lost a child in any circumstance, therefore I prayed this would never happen to me.

At the start of my second year of school nursing I spent the first few weeks preparing staff with emergency first aid kits and teaching CPR to a few staff members. The new students in our elementary school had yet to figure out that they could visit the school nurse and get all the love and attention they might need and possibly a call home to their mom. Therefore, I had not been very busy on this Friday afternoon during the second week of school.

At around 2 p.m. that day the office staff called the clinic stating that I was needed for a student on the playground. I grabbed my emergency first aid kit and hurriedly took off. Arriving on the playground I saw that the first graders had been eating ice cream and having their afternoon recess. I also saw a small blonde-headed boy lying flat on his back with a teacher at his side. She was visibly upset. I asked, "What happened?" The teacher said the child told a boy he was playing with that he didn't feel well, and as the boy ran to tell the teacher, the child collapsed to the ground.

My initial assessment told me the child was not breathing. As I started the ABC's of CPR, I asked God for the strength and wisdom to help this child; he was lying so peaceful and serene. The teachers rushed the first graders off the playground as I began chest compressions and another teacher called 911. The paramedics arrived within minutes and began to intubate and defibrillate. We continued CPR as we loaded him into the ambulance. I took his tiny hand as he was lifted into the ambulance, squeezed and kissed it, saying, "You're going to be okay."

The principal and I followed the ambulance to the hospital arriving first to the emergency room. We waited in hopes to hear that the child was okay. The child's mother and her friend arrived shortly wanting to know what happened. We told her that Michael had been playing on the playground when he collapsed and stopped breathing. "Could he have been bee stung?" she asked. I told her I didn't think so, but that I wasn't sure what had happened. We sat anxiously in a small room and waited for news on his condition.

Eventually, a doctor walked in the room and knelt down by the mother. Taking her hand, he said, "I'm sorry, we did all we could do." I'll never forget her words as she said, "How fitting of Michael to go on the playground. He was so full of life." She cried softly until her husband arrived and received the sad news. Michael's father asked to see the child. I can't remember the exact words of the father's prayer as we stood around this precious little boy lying on a stretcher but I do remember that it was the most beautiful prayer. He said that Michael was a precious gift to their family and that now he had been called home.

My greatest fear had come true, but because of these two wonderful parents' show of faith and courage in the midst of tragedy, I knew I would find the strength to continue my profession. Yes, I would go on to have strength to serve the children, know the children, teach, touch, heal and love the children. I prayed that I would have courage and wisdom to hear silent cries for help, see when a parent needed support and have a gentle and skilled hand that would heal and cure those in need.

As my heart was breaking for this family, I asked why such a tragedy could occur. Then I begin to ask, *how can I make a difference and make this world a better place?*

The answer came as I realized that God works through people like Michael's parents. They had shown through their faith and actions that we must have the courage and faith to continue. My prayer now is for all children to have a loving and courageous family as Michael did and that we all have the same strength and courage to make this world a better place for children.

Eventually, doctors determined that Michael died from a condition called Long Q-T syndrome. His mother, brother and sister take medication to prevent this electrical dysfunction from occurring in their hearts. Scientists and doctors have now determined that an AED (Automated External Defibrillator) can assist in preventing these types of untimely deaths. Schools and many public places are now equipped with these life-saving devices.

My lesson is that in spite of preparation and prayers our higher power is always in control. Even when our prayers aren't answered as we wish, we as nurses must have the strength to persevere. I hope as school nurses our actions reflect our faith and that we will be instruments for a better world for children.

To contact Jeannie Edwards, send an email to jedwards@dawson.k12.ga.us.

Fighting For What You Believe

By Cynthia S. Perry, CPNP, MSN

The phone call came in that morning and it wasn't good news. The city budget was being voted on by our City Council in 24 hours. Included in this budget was the elimination of some school nurse positions. I was one of the supervisors of this department and was told that the cuts were inevitable. Our city health department provided the school nurses to a large intercity public school district, and already our human resources were stretched well beyond the recommended ratio of one nurse to every 750 students. I've worked in the school nursing field for over 16 years, both in direct care and management, and I was well aware of the city's needs. The reality of the job is that there are never enough resources to accomplish the many needs of our schools and now we were going to have even less to work with.

The other supervisor and I met and talked that morning about how we would handle the situation. We considered which nurses we could juggle and which schools would no longer get nursing services. We also talked about how we could keep morale up for a dedicated staff that gave so much to the children of our community: hardly ever taking lunch without interruption, putting together programs on their own time and spending their own money to buy things for kids who needed so much. Many were making less money than they made before coming to us and put everything they had into their job because they believed in the value of a child. All morning we tried to come up with plans to deal with the impending situation, but neither of our hearts were in it. The truth was that we wanted to fight for our budget, but we were told that it was futile to do so.

Sometimes the strength to do what seems impossible comes in a totally unexpected way. I found strength that day while at lunch at a fast food restaurant. A young woman in her twenties was the manager of the restaurant, aptly named Angel, as I needed an angel at that point.

The young woman walked up to me and said, "Ms. Cindy, do you remember me? I just wanted you to know I'm doing good. Thank you."

I remembered the woman as a young teenage mom who came from a family with a lot of struggles. She was always getting into some type of trouble and tended to skip school as often as she came. She and I had some spirited discussions about her future and I never thought she heard what I was trying so hard for her to hear: that she deserved better. With that "thank you," I realized she had heard me in her own time. I made up my mind right then and there that we were going to fight and somehow we were going to win.

We sought community support for school nurses and it came in well beyond our expectations. In less than 24 hours, our city council members' offices were inundated with thousands of telephone calls from principals, teachers and parents on the need for school nurses. Our budget wasn't cut that year and within the next year it was actually increased.

Sometimes you have just got to believe that people are going to hear what you are trying so hard to say. This time they did, and the children of our community won.

To contact Cynthia Perry, send an email to aazzmmpp@aol.com.

A New Profile in Courage

By Kathy Borniger, RN

I believe that as school nurses we bring many things to our jobs. All of our experiences as individuals, family members, parents and nurses contribute to our daily tasks. While sometimes overwhelming, our work is consistently rewarded by the strength we draw from the children in our care. One of my favorite stories is about a boy named Alex who always gave his very best.

Alex was in second grade at my school, a Catholic institution with about 720 students from pre-kindergarten through eighth grade. He struggled academically since kindergarten and was diagnosed with severe dyslexia the year before. As the school curriculum advanced and became more difficult, Alex struggled even more. Several times he became overwhelmed as the day progressed, causing his teacher and I to agree to allow him to come to my office and "chill out" for five or 10 minutes when necessary. When in my office, he would rest quietly or we would talk. After a few minutes, when he was ready, he would take a deep breath, get a drink of water and return to the classroom.

In March of that year, Alex's mom came to my office with a message. The night before, as she and Alex were talking about Lenten resolutions, he told her three things that he planned to do:

- Try harder in school (of course, he always tried his hardest).
- Give up chocolate (he knew that this was going to be very difficult because he really loved it).

- Give up Mrs. Borniger—me! (He would try to be strong and remain in the classroom as much as possible.)

In all my years of nursing, I don't believe I ever had a finer compliment. I ranked right up there with chocolate in the eyes of a child. I couldn't have been more proud.

Alex worked very hard during Lent. With the extra activities associated with preparing for First Communion on top of his academic challenges, he displayed great perseverance.

Alex transferred to another school the next year that was better equipped to meet his needs. I continue to hear good things about him, and he continues to come to this parish for religion classes. In the last year, I learned that Alex's father needed a bone marrow transplant and that Alex was the best match. He went through the difficult procedure and, from what I've heard, his father is doing well. With Alex's marrow and blood cells running through his veins, how could he not be doing well?

Sometimes it takes a child to show us the best in ourselves. Alex will always be my hero because of his courage and quiet perseverance. Someone once said that courage is the quiet voice at the end of the day that says, "I will try again tomorrow." That sums up Alex.

To contact Kathy Borniger, send an email to kborniger@yahoo.com.

Reaching the Top

By Wendy LaMonde, RN, BSN

As a school nurse for the last three years I've had the privilege of sharing in the lives of students and their families. I have two children but, since becoming a school nurse, it is as though I have 300 because I care about each and every student as if they were my own.

The story I am most fond of is about a 10-year-old boy who touched my life in a very special way. This student was diagnosed with a degenerative eye disease. Shortly after this diagnosis, he learned that he had a tumor in his brain. The combination of these diagnoses caused him a great deal of emotional and physical pain which included frequent headaches. Through this horrible time in his life he chose me to confide in and to lean on.

As part of the student's fifth grade year his class participates in a hike up to the top of a mountain. Given his medical situation and the relationship we developed, I was chosen to accompany him on the trip. I had countless mixed emotions about going but ultimately decided to rise to the challenge.

The hike up the mountain was difficult for both of us. The way up was complicated by many headaches requiring frequent stops. At one point the adults in the group recommended that the student and I stay behind and rest so he could recuperate. He would not hear of it and loudly expressed his need to be part of the group and continue up the mountain.

Four long hours later we reached our destination. His teacher told me that getting to the top of the mountain was like being on top of the world. In many ways it was, because it was such a triumph for both me and the student.

I feel honored that I had the opportunity to share this experience with this student. He taught me a lesson in perseverance. Many times I wanted to give up because the hike was too difficult. However, I looked to him for strength and inspiration and was able to keep going and reach the top.

Although it may be a long and bumpy road for this student, I am gratified that I have been chosen to travel with him.

To contact Wendy LaMonde, send an email to w_lmonde@sau9.org.

A Child's Logic

By Betty Daniels, RN

I have been a school nurse for seven years and love the job. The rewards of working with children are never ending, and at times I also feel rewarded from working with parents. One of our biggest challenges, and I am sure all school nurses would agree, is the dreaded head lice. I have found that parents know everything there is to know about lice and have tried just about every treatment imaginable.

Last December I had the misfortune of being diagnosed with breast cancer and had to limit my visits to the school while undergoing chemotherapy. This was very hard for me to do because I love being around children and listening to their stories. When describing the things children say, people always remark, "out of the mouths of babes." I found this all so true one morning while visiting my clinic.

It was medication time so I knew I would see a lot of the children that I hadn't seen in months. I was excited about this, as I had grown attached to them. After many students had come and gone I was sitting in my office and in walked Summer. Summer is a delight and always full of questions and suggestions. As she looked at my head covered with a baseball cap, she said, "You shaved your hair, didn't you?"

Not wanting to make a big deal about the cancer I took the ball cap off and said, "Yep. How do you like it?" She remarked that she thought it looked "pretty cool." I gave Summer her usual candy-treat and she went out the door. Just then she popped her head back in, looked me straight in the face and said, "You had lice, didn't you?"

To that I had to laugh. Even though I have been very fortunate and never had the critters in my seven years of nursing, I will always smile and remember Summer's little remark as I watch my hair slowly grow back.

To contact Betty Daniels, send an email to bettyrn1@earthlink.net.

The Bicycle

By Susan Hightower, MSN, ARNP, FNP-C

On September 11th the world stood still for all Americans as we watched the televisions' view of the catastrophe of the World Trade Center. For the school system at Fort Campbell, Kentucky, it meant jeeps with armed soldiers guarding our schools, parents and children worrying they would have to go to war, fear in everyone's eyes, and long lines lasting hours to get into the school's gates.

Being an assertive person who thinks at 40 I can do what I did at 16, I borrowed my son's bike and helmet and decided to park across the street from the gate and ride my bike to work. I could bypass all the traffic and felt that because I was the school nurse, "they needed me."

The trip to work went pretty well. The worst thing I did was drop a soda at the foot of a soldier, which almost cost me my life. I felt very proud riding the mile or two and all the teachers thought I did so well.

At the end of the day I was riding back to my car and enjoying the sunshine. On the way down a hill to my car, I hit a bump, lost control and went across the pavement in front of oncoming traffic. Skinned knees and arms were the worst of my physical injuries; when I looked at the bustling traffic and realized that I had a large audience, I wanted to crawl under the pavement!

The next day I had to wear a dress to keep anything from rubbing the Band aides on my knees. There were, of course, inevitable questions and embarrassment, but I went on with my day. During the afternoon hours, there was a precious little girl who came in for an illness. She asked me what I did to my knees, and I told her. She looked up at me very seriously and said, "I think you need your daddy to put your training wheels back on your bicycle." I very seriously said, "I think you're right." I gave her a hug and sent her on her way. She was a bright star on an otherwise depressing day.

People ask me all the time why I would want to be a full time school nurse when there are so my other things I could do. This young lady says it all! God gave us children so we remember our place in the world!

To contact Susan Hightower, send an email to SHightow@fced.org.

I Believe I Can Fly

By Caroline Champion, RN, MSN, CSN

James was a fourth grader who lived with an oxygen tank as his constant companion. He would either be tethered to a tank in the classroom or to a portable pack he carried in his backpack. He was born with a right diaphragmatic hernia: a genetic disorder that produced a hole in his diaphragm and caused his lungs to deteriorate. When he came to our school he had already undergone seven surgeries. Because only one of his lungs was functioning, he had to be on oxygen 24 hours a day. His family moved to our area because of the proximity to a major children's hospital that could perform lung transplant surgery. His mother carried a pager and was ready to leave in an instant if a compatible set of lungs became available.

In spite of everything that James had endured, he was always upbeat. He loved to sing and really liked Shania Twain. His rendition of her songs could be heard throughout the school. He almost always had an infectious smile on his face and was an inspiration to his classmates.

James had endured so much in his young life and was now facing imminent, life-threatening surgery. His teacher and I decided to organize a James P. Day. We opted for February 14 as the day of the rally and held it in our gymnasium. We chose Valentine's Day because it was the holiday that expressed heart and love. We wanted everyone to show the "heart" they had for James.

City officials, school board members, the Saint Louis Cardinals' mascot, Fredbird, two Saint Louis Rams cheerleaders, a U. S. Representative and all of the staff and students in the district attended.

We sold t-shirts that everyone wore and helped raise $5,000 for a fund set up for James. The backs of the shirts were printed with the words, "I Believe I Can Fly," from a popular song. We chose those words because that's what he believed. It was his motto. The rally received extended media coverage not only from newspapers, but television as well. James was the recipient of many gifts and accolades, but the visual support of 1,000 children and adults all wearing "I Believe I Can Fly" t-shirts was a boost to his spirits.

Four months after the rally, James underwent a six-hour surgery and received two healthy lungs. Within hours of being removed from the ventilator, he was sitting up, walking, and watching videos of his favorite singer, Shania Twain.

The overall one-year survival rate for lung-transplant patients is 77 percent. Thankfully for James, he has beaten the odds. It has now been three years since the surgery, and he is thriving. His teacher and I would like to think that our efforts helped make a difference in the success of James' surgery, but actually I believe his outlook and perseverance motivated us. His cheerful attitude in the face of adversity made us see that our minor annoyances were petty. We wanted to show James the "heart" that everyone had for him, but instead he showed us.

To contact Caroline Champion, send an email to cchamp@stclair.k12.il.us.

The Mighty Seven

By Susan E. Smith, RN, BSN, MA

In school nursing, it's often a toss-up as to whether you impact a child's life or they impact yours. In the case of The Mighty Seven, I was definitely the winner. They defined my role from the beginning of our relationship and continually helped me "raise the bar".

In opening a new school a number of years ago I had several classes of self-contained special education students defined at the time as educable mentally handicapped. Many of these students had multiple medical diagnoses along with their learning challenges. From the beginning, the primary class bonded like glue. They ranged in age from six to eight and created a social group that rivaled any I've ever seen. From first grade on, they had slumber parties and sleepovers, were involved in Special Olympics and were each other's cheering section. It was a joy to witness the unconditional friendship these seven kids had for each other and anyone who entered their world. They embraced the world with joy and celebrated every milestone with hugs and laughter, and shared heartaches with hugs and tears. I remember well the day in fourth grade that one of these kids named Matt came bursting into my office proudly waving a piece of paper. He had written his name independently and had completed his simple addition problems flawlessly. That was cause for celebration!

Days with substitute teachers created a special stress for these students. They were undeniably loyal to their teachers. Early one Friday morning, the office area heard a commotion that was unbelievable. I went to my door only to be grabbed by 14 little hands. They were simultaneously trying to tell me something at the top of their voices, making incoherent noise. They all had speech difficulties and were difficult to understand in the best of circumstances. Despite how small they all were, they pushed and pulled until I headed in the direction of their classroom. (Later the secretary told me the substitute teacher called her in a panic because she lost her class. "Don't worry," she responded. "The nurse found them.")

Down the stairs, around the corner and into the classroom they pulled me while chattering non-stop at a loud and fast rate—I didn't understand a word of it. Straight to the hamster cage we went. The hamster was having babies and they wanted me to help!

One voice came through loud and clear: "The daddy is eating the babies!" I grabbed a spiral notebook and separated the father from the mother and babies. The father was mad and hissing at me. Seven little sets of eyes were watching me with confidence. They did not seem to know that nursing school did not prepare me for hamster midwifery and were sure I could rise to the occasion. What an experience!

About a year later, the crew bolted into my health office once again—minus one. By now I could understand their speech better and clearly understood that one of the mighty seven, Alex, was in trouble. As they pulled me into the music room, I saw Alex lying on the floor like he was in a casket. He was stretched out rigid with his hands folded over his chest, eyes closed tightly and lips pursed while the substitute teacher hovered over him wringing her hands.

"What happened?" I asked as I kneeled by him.

"I think he stood up too fast and fainted," the substitute answered.

"Alex, are you OK?" I asked as I checked his pulse. He peered at me under one lash and I could see an almost imperceptible nod of his head. I realized that he was embarrassed that he had fallen in front of someone he did not know. I asked if the teacher would take the class into the adjacent room for a minute, but Alex's friends were not about to leave him. Finally, the teacher left the classroom and after making sure that only his friends and I were present, he got up and came into my office. He did not open his eyes until he was in my office so nobody could see him, and ended up being fine. One thing I learned from these special friends was that if they could not see you, you could not see them. Not a bad rule for life!

Another strength of The Mighty Seven was problem-solving. They had their own pace for all of life's activities and no schedule in the world was going to change it. Austin took his time in the bathroom, and his bathroom visits often coincided with after-lunch recess. The paraeducator was struggling because it took him so long and the others wanted to be on the playground. "No problem," I said. "He can use the bathroom in my office and I will take him to the playground when he is ready."

For a few days, all went as planned. Then one day Austin concerned me by the amount of time he was in the bathroom. Fifteen minutes passed and the door was still locked. "Austin, do you need help?" I hollered though the bathroom door. "No," he responded. Twenty minutes passed, the door was still locked. I hollered through the bathroom door, "Austin, do you need help?" "No," he responded. "If you don't open the door I will need to get a key and open it," I said. "No," was his response. I went to get the key. Just as I returned to open the door, out came Austin. Every pocket of his jeans, shirt and coat were packed full of toilet paper and it was trailing to the floor.

"Why do you have toilet paper in your pockets?" I asked. "Out at home," was his response. I could barely contain my grin. Austin's mother was a good friend by now and I knew I needed to alert her before the clothes were put in the laundry, so I called and shared the story. "Just a minute," she said. She returned to the phone a few minutes later and while laughing said, "His bathroom is out of toilet paper!"

Watching these special kids grow up with their unique challenges was rewarding. Two boys were able to get jobs at the local grocery store as sackers as part of their vocational education. They would grin ear to ear when I was able to get in one of the lines they were serving. Matt was determined to be a cashier despite doubts that he had the skills and ability to manage money and work with the public. They were wrong. He convinced the manager to give him an opportunity to try; assuring him that he could count money. I think I must have been one of his first customers. He rang up my bill while carrying on an appropriate conversation. I think even his teachers were surprised. He ended up being one of the best cashiers in the store's history.

After eight years, I was transferred to another school in our district. I had been there about two years when one afternoon I heard a commotion in the outer office. "Where's Mrs. Smith?" a voice boomed. I headed toward the office to see what was happening. There was Matt, all two hundred and twenty pounds of him. He picked me up in a big bear hug and said, "I went to school to find you and they said you moved. I've been looking all over for you. *I got my driver's license!*" Sure enough, this determined little boy who struggled to learn his alphabet and numbers had managed to succeed! By working hard he was able to get a job and the coveted driver's license. And even after all that time, he went looking for his school nurse to celebrate.

To contact Susan Smith, send an email to ssmithsn@hotmail.com.

The "Special"-Ed Student

By Mari Shooks, RN

I've been a school nurse at a K–4 elementary school for nineteen years. Five years ago a special education student named Angelo entered my school as a first grader. I truly enjoy all my little ones, but it was love at first sight for me when I met this boy. This child had huge brown eyes, a winning smile and a personality to match. I saw him twice a day for medication administration and we had our own little private jokes and secrets. It wasn't long before I thought Angelo had as much affection for me as I had for him. He stayed with us through the fourth grade.

Our school holds a small "flying up" ceremony when the students are leaving us for their middle school career. About a month before this ceremony was to take place, Angelo's special education teacher approached me and asked if I was planning to attend the celebration. I wasn't sure if I could attend at that point but asked if she needed help with anything. She replied that Angelo had written a story that he was going to read at the ceremony and that the story was about me. With tears in my eyes I assured the teacher that I would cancel my other plans and certainly be there.

The big night came and the teacher asked me to sit in the front of the auditorium so that I could be Angelo's point of focus. I wanted him to be successful so I was willing to do whatever was needed. When it was Angelo's turn and he was called to the dais, he got up out of his seat and instead of going to the microphone; he came over to my seat and presented me with a box of Kleenex. All of his classmates were laughing because they were "in" on this part of the presentation. Then he went to the microphone and read the following composition:

"My best friend at Windham Center School is my nurse, Mrs. Shooks. She is my favorite person because she always makes me happy by being nice to me and giving me hugs. She missed me when I had to stay home because I had an ear infection. She is my favorite person because she takes my blood pressure and reminds me to take my medicine. I will miss her when I go to the middle school. She doesn't want me to go to the middle school because she is going to miss me too much. I hope my new nurse is like Mrs. Shooks. Mrs. Shooks is a wonderful nurse."

By this time I was sobbing in front of students, parents, the superintendent, board of education members, my principal and teachers. I really was grateful for the box of tissues he had just given me! The hug we shared after his presentation was the best hug we had ever shared. Later, his teacher told me that Angelo had composed his story several weeks before the ceremony and had been practicing his recitation since. It was also his idea to present me with the tissue because he knew I would cry.

Occasionally I get up to the middle school to see my friend and tell him how much I miss him. He assures me that his new nurses aren't as wonderful as me and that he still loves me best. He says he's growing up now and doesn't want to come back to elementary school—not even for a visit. I'm not sure I'll ever find another student who is as "special" as this student.

To contact Mari Shooks, send an email to mshooks@windham.k12.ct.us.

Courage for the Future

By Sally Schoessler, RN, SNT

My elementary school has always gone out of their way to make National School Nurse Day a special day for me. On that special day, there are often flowers, stuffed animals and posters that create a festive atmosphere in my office. My favorite part of the day has always been the pile of colorful handmade cards from individual students. Last year, two particular cards really stood out for me.

Jon, the smallest and most quiet boy in the fourth grade, stayed behind when his class came by to drop off the cards that they made for me, and told me, "I didn't bring my card yet, it's not finished. I'll bring it to you before the end of the day." I told him that I appreciated the work he was putting into the card and I would look forward to seeing him later.

It was nearly the end of the day when a beaming Jon stopped by to see me. He said that I must wait until after he left to read his card. I thanked him and paused until he turned the corner and was back to his classroom. I then opened the card.

The front of the card was a detailed pencil drawing of the school building and read, "It must take courage to be a school nurse." I slowly opened the card to see that the inside contained a picture of a nurse surrounded by children with the words: "Because everyone is always counting on you." I later told Jon that his card helped me to find my courage.

Another student named Adam gave me a card that year that brought me to tears. Adam had a particularly difficult life. He was part of a fractured family and lived in a household where no two people had the same last name. He had an assortment of mental health issues and by age 10 had two therapists and a variety of medication to keep him going on a daily basis. My one goal was to make him smile when he came to see me for his medication. As Adam came to see me on School Nurse Day, he said, "I left my card at home. I'll bring it tomorrow."

This routine went on for three days. On the fourth day, Adam produced a simple, wrinkled card illustrated with a red cross on the front with my name misspelled below. It had a dark stain in the corner and was slightly torn. He proudly said, "Read the inside. I really meant what I said."

It simply read: "You heal my future."

A Bus Stop Tragedy

By Karen K. Frecker, RN

Being a school nurse is such a wonderful experience—sometimes I feel like I'm on a roller coaster ride with the many ups and downs of this profession. This story is about a resilient elementary student who saw her stepfather die of a heart attack at her school bus stop.

This was a tragic accident for an adult to see, let alone a first grader. An ambulance took her stepfather to the hospital after he was pronounced dead at the bus stop. As you can imagine, it was very difficult for this child to go back to school and she definitely did not want to go to her bus stop again.

A few days after the funeral I made a home visit to the child's house to see what I could do to help the child and her family, and organized counseling sessions. Although the student began to come to school again, she was not ready to get back on the school bus.

I met with the child's teacher and arranged for the student to come to the nurse's office at least once a week to talk one-on-one. The student immediately felt comfortable enough to talk to me about her stepfather's death and after a short period of time was able to ride the bus again. Each week she rode the bus she would get an extra incentive. At the beginning of each day the student would get off the bus and come straight to my office, hug me, smile and then go on to class. Children are such resilient individuals.

To contact Karen Frecker, send an email to freckek@cpsboe.k12.oh.us.

IV

Easing the Pain of Troubled Children

"We have a duty to feed the souls of children longing for love and attention. This is as important for future generations as a good education in academics."

—Author of **The Girl Who Cried Wolf**
(name withheld to ensure confidentiality)

School Anxiety

By Muriel Luther, RN, BSN

Chris was new to our school that year. I received a report stating that he had not attended school for over one year and instead had been receiving home-schooling for unknown reasons. I contacted the counselor at Chris's previous school to gain further information and discovered that she and the staff had suggested home-schooling as a last resort when nothing else seemed to be effective. She said that Chris became increasingly anxious in class and developed severe headaches and altered breathing that caused him to spend most of each school day in the counselor's or the nurse's office. He was not benefiting from being at school and home-teaching was therefore ordered by his primary physician and psychiatrist. This was about to change.

All involved—parents, doctors, counselors, teachers and nurses—decided that Chris needed to return to school. A new school was chosen to avoid potential embarrassment associated with Chris having to face peers who knew his history.

Chris's mother brought him into my office at the start of school and requested that medication be administered during the school day. He impressed me as a polite sixth grader who was well-spoken. I later was informed that he was quite a bright student who received "straight A's" and was inclined to be a perfectionist. Both Chris and his mom spoke of his hesitancy to return to school but realized it was a necessity. The question I asked myself was how, as a school nurse, I could help this happen. The answers were unclear. I assured both Chris and his mother that we would do our best to help him. I started by attaining permission from his very cooperative mother to speak with his doctors.

On his first day of school, Chris remained in class for a part of first period. About halfway into the class I witnessed the anxiety that I heard about. With clenched fists, a red face, tense muscles, making loud groaning sounds and with his head down, he was brought to me crying. "I can't do it, I can't do it," he said. We were unable to resolve Chris's headache/anxiety that day and his mother eventually came for him.

Days two, three and four and many more followed a similar pattern until Chris was not able to remain in class for even thirty minutes. We quickly arranged a meeting which included his mom, the home school teacher, his doctor via telephone and involved school personnel (counselor, psychologist, RSP, vice principal and myself). We began with his physician who assured me that he needed to return to school as soon as we got a workable plan in place. Creating a workable plan was not an easy task. I approached the medical issues: Does the medication work? Are his headaches relieved with PRN medications? Has Chris expressed what seemed to benefit him most? As a group we probed his interests, his strengths and his anxiety escapes. I felt that we could potentially utilize his academic successes to decrease his tension. Together we devised a progressive plan that essentially required Chris to take "baby steps" toward lengthening his ability to stay in school. A portion of the plan involved attending class (two periods at the beginning of the day), while another portion required him to act as a reading tutor to primary grade children, one-on-one.

We implemented our plan and made changes as needed. The counselor spent parts of many mornings sitting in class with Chris offering encouraging words and support. I spent extended periods alone with Chris talking, encouraging and probing for key insight into his dilemma. We also had his psychologist visit his classroom and make suggestions to our plan. Never did we suggest to Chris that an alternative was to return to home-schooling.

A determined principal, a wise counselor, a dedicated staff, cooperative parents, understanding classmates and myself all worked together to achieve a successful outcome for Chris. Words cannot express the feeling of accomplishment felt by all, especially Chris, when it became evident that home-schooling was no longer necessary. He became a vital part of school life and maintained a reputation as an excellent student.

When Chris graduated from eighth grade it was a time of reflection. It was a reminder of events, progress, growth and successes acknowledged by both students and staff. It was also a time for Chris to reflect on how far he had come and look forward with confidence knowing he could overcome the most difficult of obstacles.

I am thankful as a school nurse to have had a small part in Chris's successful school experience. Situations such as this are a reminder of why I love my job and the many opportunities it provides me to make a difference in lives.

If you would like to contact Muriel Luther, send an email to mluther@lbusd.k12.ca.us.

Mark

By Barbara Berndt, RN

A depressed, withdrawn, freshman student named Mark began coming to the clinic almost immediately after the school year started. His two-to-three time per week visits frequently ended with his wanting to go home. His counselor from middle school informed me that Mark visited his office on a daily basis and these visits usually ended with Mark in tears.

I subsequently found out that Mark had been involved in a very traumatic incident during sixth grade where he was accidentally shot. He had missed a year of Middle School due to his gun shot wound and the effects of the trauma persisted.

It was obvious from Mark's first visit that he did not want to be in school. As the days, months and year progressed, his attitude and attendance didn't improve a great deal. I did my best to encourage him, but he usually started crying and his mother would allow him to come home.

During his junior year, his mother decided to make me the "bad guy." She insisted that I be the disciplinarian by refusing his requests to go home and making him stay in school. When I applied this approach, Mark became angry with me and gave me no choice but to lecture him sternly. These lectures did not deter him from coming back to the clinic.

Happily, Mark graduated at the end of four years and, although his grades were far from stellar, he received his diploma.

Mark has returned to visit several times since graduating and always greets me with a big hug. During one of his last visits he told me he wished his grades and attendance were better. He also said that he wished he would have listened more to the advice I gave him.

I haven't seen Mark recently, but I remember his last visit. He was no longer a withdrawn, nervous, depressed teen, but a self confident, smiling young man. While he has found employment and works steadily, he also plans to apply to EMT School in the near future. He said that being an EMT was his life-long dream.

By saying thanks, Mark made my oftentimes hectic, tumultuous and harried job worthwhile.

The Eyes of Savannah

The author's name has been omitted to ensure that the identities of the individuals in this story remain confidential.

Savannah was one of the most beautiful children I had ever seen. She was one of those kids that capture the hearts of the school staff. She was always bright, smiling and helpful. She was never a problem.

One of the security staff members brought Savannah to me one day because they were concerned. The beauty of Savannah's expressive brown eyes was marred by a purple bruise over her right eye. I was told that two weeks earlier it had been her left eye that was discolored.

Savannah's explanation for the bruising was that she fell. She was always falling she stated. She told this story in a way that sounded as if she was reciting something that someone told her to say. She explained her fall without expression, fact by fact, never faltering in her story telling. Too often I have seen brave little children tell such stories to protect those they love despite their faults.

As we talked, Savannah told me her parents often drank and then began to fight in a way that frightened her and her siblings. So this courageous child, Savannah, at just seven years old, would embrace her younger sister in her arms and wipe her tears. She would take her into their bedroom, hide in the closet and close their door. She would sing songs and tell her stories to protect her from the yelling, hitting and crying. But who was there to assuage Savannah's fears?

The yelling ended, but Savannah knew the violence wouldn't stop there. Her dad left but her mom was drunk and upset. Upset because maybe Savannah, from her mother's perspective, did something to set daddy off. The mother would then hit Savannah.

Savannah, in her wisdom at the ripe old age of seven, told me that her mother really didn't mean to hurt her. She said that her mother always cried after hitting her and would tell her she was sorry and say how much she loved her. "Because daddy hurt mommy," Savannah expressed, "mommy had to hurt somebody else."

In those beautiful, brown, expressive eyes marred by a bruise, this child saw the truth of her situation. That night I went home and hugged my children tight to me and later, when I was alone, I cried. I cried for Savannah's mother who couldn't save herself or her children. I cried for Savannah's sister that she needed to be protected. But mostly I cried for Savannah, whose eyes had to see such truths.

A Thank You From the Heart

By Katheryn M. Rowell, RN, BSN, CSN, MS

In my seventeen years of school nursing, many children have left a lasting impression on me. The one who I believe has touched me the most is a student I will refer to as "J.B."

I first met J.B. when he began sixth grade at the middle school where I was working. He carried, among other things, a diagnosis of ADHD and came to the nurse's office each day for medication. There were also family issues impacting J.B.'s education. These issues exploded when he reached eighth grade and, one night during that school year, he overdosed on a bottle of whiskey and was taken to the hospital in serious condition.

When he returned to school, there was an IEP meeting where J.B.'s mother told about his stay in the hospital. While still under the influence of the alcohol he consumed, a nurse came in to take care of him. Thinking she was his school nurse, he said, "Mrs. R, why are you here so late? I really love you, Mrs. R. I'm so glad you are here." J.B. sheepishly related this same information to me one day in my office later in the school year.

On the last day of school, J.B. came in to say good-bye and we chatted about his future at high school. He walked to the door to leave, turned around and quietly said, "Thank you for being my school nurse."

It was a touching moment that definitely deserved a hug before he left the middle school for that walk into the future.

If you would like to contact the Katheryn Rowell, send an email to krowell@wcasd.k12.pa.us.

The Elevator Boy

By Fay Little, RN

My first assignment as a school nurse was at a very small and nurturing continuation high school. While most students at this high school were not exactly the most motivated, there was a boy who seemed to truly want to be there to study and graduate. His name was Edmund.

But Edmund had a problem: he was afraid of climbing the stairs. When approaching stairs, he would break into a cold sweat, his heart would race, and he would become light headed.

Since this was a two-story school and some of his classes were upstairs, the principal felt obligated to allow him to take the elevator even though it was a downright nuisance. The security guard, already quite busy, had to unlock the elevator door for Edmund as many as four times a day. The nurturing staff did this without questioning and without documentation for any real health problem.

Enter the school nurse who can't just let things be. I requested a medical exam to investigate any underlying physiological reason. Everything was negative. He had gone to a therapist in the past for other problems and was prescribed anti-anxiety medication. He refused to take it because it made him feel funny. The elevator rides continued.

I actually lacked confidence to boldly declare that the boy may simply be having panic attacks that would be easy to get a handle on. Meanwhile, the staff was afraid he would collapse and sue everyone. I secretly wanted to say to Edmund that he should just *get over it!* I knew what I really needed was a systemic approach to counsel him on how to deal with his fear. A method had to exist somewhere.

Then, towards the end of the school year, I received a newsletter for school nurses with a short article about dealing with panic attacks. I copied it and sent it to Edmund.

When school reconvened in September, I forgot all about the Elevator Boy. Months went by and I didn't even think of the boy and his fear of stair climbing until I saw him once again when he reported for an IEP. I called him in for the routine assessment and he thanked me for sending the article. He had been able to climb stairs since September.

If you would like to contact Fay Little, send an email to flittle@gusd.net.

The Girl Who Cried Wolf

The author's name has been omitted to ensure that the identities of the individuals in this story remain confidential.

Julie's mother is a doctor at a women's clinical research center and her father is a surgeon. Her parents have plenty of money to send her to an elite private school for the best possible education and small class size, ensuring individual attention to her scholastic needs. She attends before and after school programs regularly, arriving at 7:30 a.m. and leaving at 5:00 p.m. She participates in sports programs and special after-school classes often.

This scenario is quite different from the public school domain where middle class and underprivileged families mix to survive in this hard economy. At our school we have very few children with physical disabilities or developmental delays. Our students have to pass an IQ test at ages four or five to remain in this highly academic program. Social skills are also a consideration and children with little motivation and low confidence in the classroom are weeded out regularly. Despite these strict student admission guidelines, to say that we don't have any special needs children would be misleading to say the least. We have a very high rate of asthma, allergies, and depression—among other things.

The school counselor is a very busy person, as am I, the health officer. The problems that stem from lack of parental contact, the pressure of a fast paced schedule, high academic expectations, and home models of high-end careers are tremendous. Many of our parents are in the medical field, and sometimes children try to get their parents attention by getting sick or hurt. It is a subconscious action for some, while for others it is a highly contrived act of desperation.

Julie visits the health office every day, as do some of the others. It becomes my job to try to discern real ailments from the imagined and empower these students to focus on healthy thinking. When communicating illnesses to the parents I often get the response: "Can't you just give her some Tylenol?" or, "I can't leave work, can she stay there with you?" or, "I'll call the nanny to pick her up."

One week the need to be hurt was very strong in Julie. She came to the health office on Monday to tell me that she had fallen over the weekend and could not move her left arm at all. She explained that it hurt to bend and she needed a sling. I examined her arm thoroughly and saw no signs of pain. Her arm had no inflammation or redness. She stuck to her claim with tears welling in her eyes, but I sent her to class without the sling. Later I observed her playing on the monkey bars at recess.

The next day she came to school with a sling on. She had a big smile on her face and had a happy day. At recess she took it off and played on the monkey bars. I asked her if her arm was better and she said it still hurt a little, but not very much.

On Wednesday she truly got hurt. Some of her friends came running into the Office saying, "Cathy, come quickly, Julie fell and she can't get up. Hurry!"

I ran outside with them to the monkey bars. Julie was lying on her left side crying. The recess assistant looked worried and said he was afraid to move her. I knelt down and asked her, "What hurts the most Julie?" She said she couldn't move. She was crying hard. I took a deep breath and asked her if her leg hurt as I felt it gently. She answered, "no." I asked her if she could move her legs. She straightened them out and nodded her head—so her head was moving as well. I checked her ankles. I felt her spine and asked if her back hurt—her answer again was "no." She stopped crying.

Her left arm was still beneath her although she had straightened out somewhat. I asked about the left arm and she said it hurt. I gently reached under her back and very slowly laid her flat, keeping her arm against her body and her head in line. She raised her head and reached across with her right arm and held onto her left arm. I asked the male TA if he would carry her to the office. He asked if I was sure we should move her and I said yes. I held her left arm immobile and supported her head as he lifted from the right—we carried her inside. She sat up with support and I continued to assess the left arm, shoulder and neck. Her left shoulder was raised and a little jutted forward. It looked like a possible dislocation or even collar bone injury. She was crying again and experiencing what looked like a little shock. I wrapped her arm to her torso to immobilize her left side, made sure she had plenty of support all around with pillows and got some ice. I covered her with a blanket and raised her feet. Her teacher came in and when I felt she was in a good position I called her mom.

Her mother sighed and told me that Julie had been pretending to be injured for two weeks. I told her that I felt this was legitimate and explained that her daughter's left shoulder was jutting forward, she could not move it, she was pale and cold, crying hard, and that she needed to see a doctor. I was told to wait another 15 minutes and keep assessing the situation, and to call her back if I still felt she needed treatment. I hung up reluctantly and consulted with Julie's teacher. We both felt she was really hurt and her mother needed to come. Julie was obviously injured, to what degree we did not know, but I was not comfortable without a doctor's examination. I called her mother back and told her that the teacher was of the same opinion as I, and that she needed to come to the school. She sighed again and told me that on Monday evening she came home to find Julie sprawled in a position at the bottom of the stairs that no one could possibly land in, saying she couldn't move, crying and holding her left arm. She said that she could find nothing wrong with Julie, but gave her a sling anyway.

As we waited for Julie's mother to arrive I spoke privately to the teacher and shared my feelings about a dysfunctional relationship between mother and daughter in regard to illness and injury. We had discussed this before, but the fact that Julie's mother gave her a sling when she was obviously pretending to be injured did not seem right to me.

Julie walked out with her mom and the diagnosis from the hospital was a strained shoulder. She came to school the next day with a sling and a big smile. I am not certain how much of the incident was drama, but if it was, Julie should win an academy award! Her mother thanked me for insisting she come. She said that she had not believed Julie was really hurt, but admitted that the hospital staff confirmed the injury as legitimate. This type of scenario is typical at the school where I work.

There is more to our jobs than the normal scrapes, bumps, colds, sand in the eyes, knocked-out teeth, occasional broken bones, peanut allergies, insect bites, and objects up the nose. We must also nurse the broken hearts, tensions, depressions and fears.

We have a duty to feed the souls of children longing for love and attention. This is as important for future generations as a good education in academics.

The Boy Who Cried Wolf

By Joyce A. Sheppard, RN

One morning early in the school year a boy from the kindergarten class walked into my office with "pains" in his lower abdomen. The child was familiar to me since he was on daily medication for ADHD and very comfortable coming to the health office. Upon initial visual assessment, he did not appear in acute distress. When asked the usual questions, he answered: yes, he had eaten his breakfast and no, he was not hungry. His temperature was normal. I sent him to the bathroom and he doubled over in "pain."

Throughout my assessment he indicated that his pain was worsening. Palpitation of the right lower quadrant seemed to produce more discomfort. He appeared to be positive for rebound tenderness. I put a call out to his mother and was awaiting her return call thinking that the child may have appendicitis since he now was lying on the cot in my office and writhing in pain.

I was then called out of the office and was just outside the door when I heard my telephone ring. As I opened the door, there was the boy standing straight upright, answering the telephone with a smile on his face, thinking that it was his mother calling to say that she would be picking him up.

His mother and I quickly agreed that the child just wanted to go home. I then had a discussion with the boy about how he could communicate his feelings about school without using the "sick excuse." After a talk about "the boy who cried wolf" and not answering other people's telephone, he returned to class. He finished the school year with no further visits to the health office except for his daily medication, screenings or to occasionally deliver messages from his teacher.

He left my school after that year. I often think about him and that incident. I like to think that something I said that day made a difference in him not becoming a frequent flyer to the nurse's office and staying in the classroom.

If you would like to contact Joyce Sheppard, send an email to JASandJMS@aol.com.

V

The Day-to-Day Life of a School Nurse

"I spent my first nine years after graduation as a critical care nurse, first in a mixed Med—Surgical Intensive Care Unit and then in a Coronary Care Unit. Then, there was a brief stint as an in-service instructor followed by several years of staff relief for an agency. I thought that I had seen just about every tough case that there ever was. School nursing would be a piece of cake—just apply Band aids and call parents... right! *I didn't have a clue."*

—Claire Vey, RN

All in a Day's Work

By Debbie Doggett, RN

The weatherman said it would reach 90 degrees today. Maybe a cloud will cover the sun. Thankfully, we sent notes home instructing parents to put sunscreen on their children before sending them off to school. Everything is set up outside. The activities look like a lot of fun! The PE teachers have been working on it for weeks. Please God, keep all the children safe and let them have a wonderful day!

The phone starts ringing.

"Susie is vomiting but really does not want to miss field day," says one parent. "Can she come? No? But she has not vomited since last night! She's not sick. She just ate too much for supper."

"I'm sorry," I reply. "Our school policy states that she will have to stay home until she has not vomited for at least 24 hours."

I look up and a teacher is standing at the clinic door with a child. "Fred told me he threw up before he came to school," the teacher states. "What should we do?"

Two other children come walking in behind them with sick slips. One of the children's parents did not put any sunscreen on her for field day. The other child has medication and a note from her mom asking me to give her child the medication at lunch. She must have forgotten to read the parent handbook which specifically states that medications are to be brought to school by a responsible adult. The other parent must not have seen the note sent home asking parents to apply sunscreen.

Suddenly, a teacher approaches me saying, "Nurse! Come quick. The custodian just cut her wrist."

I instruct the custodian to press down hard on the wound while I put on my gloves. I assure her that she will be okay as I sit her down on a chair. She turns white as a ghost and as I wash off the blood, I think to myself, *thank you Lord—that it is not an artery!* I apply a sterile pressure bandage and wrap it in gauze. I tell the secretary to get someone to take her to the emergency room to have it stitched. Before they leave I give her last minute instructions on what to do if she starts to feel faint and send her off in capable hands.

In the meantime, four more children show up. "Next!" I announce. A little girl complains of her tummy hurting. Her face looks very flushed; she was outside running. I have her drink some water and lie down to rest. I give her a warm towel to hold on her stomach. The phone rings and I have several parents calling in to report their children absent from school. The attendance sheet I ran off earlier is still lying on my desk, waiting for me to call the parents. There are only 30 children absent today. That's much better than the 60 absences we had on a single day last week!

The principal calls and asks if I filled out an accident report on the custodian and completed the necessary workman's compensation forms. I assure her I will.

Several teachers email me about absentees. My current immunization list shows three children due for immunizations this week before they can come back to school. I notify the parents and leave messages.

Just one more hour till lunch time! I decide to take a restroom break but before I leave a child walks in. According to the teacher, she has been scratching her head all morning. It turns out that she has lice for the fourth time this year. I notify her mom who insists it's the school's fault. I then email the teachers to bring their classes to the clinic so I can check every head to make sure there are no other cases. I make a note: *Don't forget to send letters to all the parents of children in those rooms notifying them of lice in their child's classroom. Also, notify the custodians to vacuum the room well and bag up all stuffed animals and play clothes for 10 days.*

Lunchtime!! Oh Good! I am starving and really need to make a trip to the bathroom! I need to draw a child's blood sugar before I go. What? She has diarrhea and you have no change of clothes? It's on her shoes too. I have the child sit down at the table, give her some books and a puzzle to work and start calling her mom to pick her up. When I am unable to reach anyone I ask the teacher to please stay and be my witness while I clean the child up. I draw the child's blood sugar, call mom because it is too low, administer two glucose tablets and walk her to the cafeteria to get lunch right away.

As I leave for my lunch a teacher comes with a child who has complained all morning and feels hot. "Can you take his temperature?" she asks. I think to myself, *why did she wait until lunchtime?* Sure enough, the child has a temperature of 103. I contact the child's mother and ask his teacher to sit with the child while I get my lunch. I eat at my desk to watch the child until his mom can pick him up.

Halfway through my meal a teacher pops her head through the door and asks if I'm almost finished with lunch. Her class is lined up in the hallway. Goodness! I almost forgot I am teaching Health today! This week I am teaching a chapter on protecting ourselves from germs. I have almost four hours of class this afternoon. In between classes I rush to the clinic to fix boo-boos, take temperatures and call moms. I must not forget to send my lesson plan for next week to the principal.

The phone rings and it is the secretary. My 2:30 p.m. appointment for medical history and vision and hearing screenings is here. The child is three years old and barely speaks. He is being evaluated for speech services. He clings to his mom and doesn't want to open his mouth. I input the child's information into the computer between phone calls about the day's absent children. It takes quite some time for the child to become relaxed enough to listen, and finally I can screen the child's hearing and vision. Just as I think he comprehends, four more children come in and need to be seen. One has cut himself with scissors, one has a bloody nose, one needs his inhaler and the other needs her Ritalin. I tell the three-year-old what a wonderful job he did, give him some stickers and let him pick a treasure from my treasure box before he leaves.

It's now 3 p.m. and almost time to go home. It's been a busy day but at least there weren't any broken bones like last field day. Another child comes to my door. The sick slip reads, "Please check bruise on neck. The child told me her daddy choked her because she would not stop crying." Finger bruises are noted so I notify Child Protection Services. I read a story to the child while we wait. She's a little frightened when the officers come to question her but is reassured when I tell her it will be okay. I think to myself, *Lord, please take care of this little one,* then give the child a hug, tell her I love her, and leave it in the hands of the authorities.

I look at the clock. If I hurry, I will have just enough time to call the Red Cross and schedule a CPR/First Aid class for the next teacher in-service day. The buses are coming and the children are lined up waiting; I walk by them all on my way back to the clinic. I hear "bye nurse" and "I love you nurse." A few children run up for a quick hug. One tells me they are putting sunscreen on every day. Another tells me she washes her hands every time she goes to the bathroom. It's a wonderful day! My heart swells with pride and love! I shout, "I love you too boys and girls! Don't forget to get a good night sleep and eat a healthy dinner!"

To contact Debbie Doggett, send an email to kendebdoggett@netzero.com.

The Hardest Job I Ever Loved

By Amy Barnes, RN, MA

It is 7 a.m. and I am mentally preparing for the day while entering my "Thursday" school. As a school nurse with an assignment of four schools (two elementary, one middle and one high school with a combined population of over 5,000 students), it takes some time to get "reprogrammed" for each new day. This is one of my elementary schools and as I walk into the office, I see the normal morning hustle and bustle. I enter the clinic and pick up my folder where my invaluable clinic assistant has placed my mail, updates regarding student concerns, the weekly report and other miscellaneous papers. I hear taps on the window as students stream by and wave on their way to class. The clinic door opens and the day begins!

In rolls one of my most medically fragile students. He is a wheelchair bound fourth grader who has a tracheostomy, continuous oxygen, and an infectious smile. He wants to tell me all about his recent fishing trip sponsored by the Make a Wish Foundation. It is great to see him so animated and full of excitement. Other students arrive with medication refills, notes from parents and clinic passes. My clinic assistant brings us both coffee and we attempt to catch up on a week's worth of information as we tend to the children's needs. Oh, the life of a school nurse: kissing boo boos and putting on Band aids—*not even close!*

I am always amazed when I talk to parents, teachers and other individuals in the community and discover how little they understand the role of the school nurse. Today's school population includes an increasing number of children with significant health problems, some of them life threatening. The nurse must be someone who can function well as an independent practitioner. Interpersonal skills and the ability to be an effective communicator are a must since the nurse is working with children, parents, medical professionals, faculty and school administrators. The nurse must also have exceptional assessment and problem solving skills since we do not have sophisticated medical technology at our immediate disposal. And on top of physical issues—the emotional and psychosocial needs of students are incredible.

Who would have thought that as a school nurse I would be involved with more emergency life saving interventions than I was in all my years as a hospital based nurse? I have often said that one day I would write a book entitled, *I Couldn't Make This Up if I Tried!* I've had a seventh grader come to my office complaining of a stomach ache—it turned out that her C-section incision was opening up. Another student came to my office bleeding profusely from his ear because a fellow student decided to cut off his earlobe for no specific reason. The list of incredible incidents is never ending. I remember telling my husband that at times I feel like I am in the Peace Corps in my own community.

As I take a sip of coffee, the clinic phone rings. The person on the other end of the phone identifies herself as an employee of the epidemiology department of our county health department. She states that a student at a high school assigned to me died in the early morning hours from bacterial meningitis. She asked that I go to the high school and find out which students may have been in close contact with the deceased student and require prophylactic antibiotic therapy. I felt my stomach twisting but instinctively my mind started with questions: Had "student X" been to the clinic the previous day and if so what were the complaints? Who were the student's teachers and how many classmates had close contact and require treatment? What did I even remember about bacterial meningitis? And, of course, I thought about how tragic this was for the student's family. The only thing I knew for certain was that I had 17 miles to put a plan together!

I quickly got my things together and threw my "office in a bag" (suitcase with wheels), into the trunk of my car and grabbed my resource books from the backseat to quickly refresh myself on the disease. I called my "Friday" school and asked to speak to the principal. I shared the news from the county health department and asked for the names of close friends of "Student X." The principal indicated that he would email only those teachers who taught the deceased student and be sure to word the email in a way that would not cause a panic. The names were to be sent to my email address. I also asked the principal to advise the guidance counselors of the situation and locate an office where I could meet quietly with students. I assured the principal that I was on my way to the school and that I would come to his office as soon as I arrived to further discuss our plan of action. I also contacted my clinic assistant at the school to let her know that I was on my way and would update her upon arrival. I then phoned my supervisor to advise her of the situation and the steps in place up to that point. She immediately assured me that she was on her way to help with this enormous and emotionally charged task.

It was now 8:20 a.m. I arrived at the high school and quickly reported to the principal. The guidance counselors soon arrived. I summarized the information I had gleaned from my medical resources as well as the information provided to me from the health department. The counselors were chiefly concerned with how the disease spread. I reinforced that since the disease is transmitted through droplets from the secretions of an infected person, unless an individual had had a recent saliva exchange (kissing, sharing food, cigarettes, etc.), the likelihood of transmission was very small. I then shared my immediate priorities which included: identifying students who may have had close contact with their deceased classmate, interviewing individuals to determine their level of exposure and informing the parents as to their child's "risk status" and treatment recommendations. This information then needed to be communicated to the epidemiology department who would determine the doses of medication required. The health department was also putting together informational letters about the disease to be sent home that afternoon with each student. They were also going to send an individual to assist with a faculty meeting scheduled after school. In addition, arrangements needed to be made for the availability of grief counselors as well as a central information center because once word got out, there would be a barrage of questions from students, parents, faculty and the press.

It was now shortly after 9 a.m. and my supervisor arrived. She spoke with the principal and other administrators as I headed to the clinic. When I shared the circumstances of this tragic situation with my assistant she was devastated. She told me that "student X" had not been to the clinic at all that week. I told her to prepare for a busy day because once news got out, there would be many students coming to the clinic for comfort and/or information.

I checked my email—the teachers had sent me the names of 17 students. I pulled their emergency cards for phone numbers to contact parents and grabbed a few boxes of Kleenex. My supervisor and I headed to our quiet space where we discussed our strategy in meeting with each student. We agreed that we needed to be compassionate while getting specific information quickly as to whether there was a risk of recent exposure to the disease. Since we had many students to meet with, we decided to take each student to the guidance counselor for additional emotional support after attaining our needed information. We took a deep breath and called the first student down.

Each session was difficult. We calmly explained that their friend had become very ill the previous evening and had passed away in the early morning hours of bacterial meningitis. We explained how the disease was transmitted and asked if they had shared any close contact with their friend within the last few days. As mentioned earlier, we needed to ascertain this information quickly before each student reacted emotionally. We then called each student's parent to give them our opinion as to whether or not their child was a candidate for prophylactic antibiotic therapy. Parents were encouraged to contact their personal physician. Most parents came to the school to comfort their child and for reassurance. Upon completion of our first round of interviews, it was determined that seven students would require medication.

During the time that we were meeting individually with the 17 students, the principal made a general announcement to school staff regarding the death of the young student. Students concerned regarding whether they had been exposed to the disease were instructed to report to the clinic. Students were also encouraged to see their guidance counselor if they required emotional support as a result of hearing this tragic news. Kids poured into the clinic and the front office in a wide range of emotional states. Again, my wonderful clinic assistant was able to provide some order to the chaos and additional grief counselors became available to assist.

Informational notices about bacterial meningitis were delivered to the school as well as the required medication permission slips. The health department informed my clinic assistant that she was to collect signed permission slips the following morning after which medication (to be delivered by the health department) could be administered.

The school day was an emotional blur and finally came to a close after which a mandatory faculty meeting was held. Again, information about how the disease is spread was shared and staff was reassured that their risk of exposure was extremely low.

All involved spent time after the faculty meeting to debrief. We discussed what worked and what did not. Our major recommendation was to communicate to teachers via email what the circumstances were and to allow each teacher to share the knowledge in a more personal way. Teachers would be notified via an announcement to check their emails. I offered to put together a protocol based on our recommendations should such a situation occur again. This protocol is now part of the *School Nurse Manual®*.

As I reflect on the events of this day, I am overwhelmed. I am convinced that what I learned from the nursing process as well as my nursing experience gave me the structure to make it through the day. My skills in assessing, critical thinking, planning, decision making, communicating, implementing and evaluating were all put to the test. As a school nurse I have learned that there is no such thing as a typical day. Days are often challenging, frustrating and rewarding at the same time. *It is the hardest job I have ever loved!*

To contact Amy Barnes, send an email to AmyB7@lee.k12.fl.us.

It's All About Learning...

By Clair Vey, RN

I began my school nursing career in a middle school. I'm not entirely sure why I changed careers midstream or why I chose a middle school. Maybe it was the lure of being at home most days when my child was at home and not having to work weekends, nights or holidays. Heaven knows it wasn't the magnificent salary. But change careers I did, and eighteen years later, I'm not sorry that I made that choice. I say that I changed careers because I spent my first nine years after graduation as a critical care nurse, first in a mixed Med—Surgical Intensive Care Unit and then in a Coronary Care Unit. Then, there was a brief stint as an in-service instructor followed by several years of staff relief for an agency. I thought that I had seen just about every tough case that there ever was. School nursing would be a piece of cake—just apply Band aids and call parents...*right!* I didn't have a clue.

I started my first day as a school nurse full of plans to make everything right for the kids in my care. I was going to quickly reorganize and restructure the health room and its operation. By the end of the day, I came to the realization that, not only was I not going to save the world, I would be lucky if I was able to dig my way out from under the massive piles of paperwork known as health records. I went home discouraged and sure that I had made a very serious career mistake. What was a critical care nurse doing in a setting without training manuals, monitors, emergency medications and a crash cart? Where was my medical direction? Where was my backup? *Where was my mind?* I did not sleep well that night and began my second day already exhausted.

As I sat at my desk surrounded by piles of documents, it suddenly occurred to me that what was needed was not the kind of care that I was used to providing. Rather, I needed to complete and organize those records, develop good triage and first aid skills and throw in a very large dose of diplomacy. I dove into that pile of records with determination while nervously anticipating the arrival of the first students of the day. I saw cuts and bruises that needed soothing and bandaging, and fearful sixth graders besieged by headaches and stomach aches who needed a different kind of TLC. I also saw wounds that were not visible in the usual manner. There were bruises and burns that were not accidental. There were too many children deeply saddened by divorce or the death of a close family member or friend. There were boys and girls so intimidated by fear of failure or being different from their peers that they no longer tried to succeed. I was absolutely astonished at the number of children who were "latch-key kids," beginning and often ending the day without parental support and attention. I saw girls starving themselves in an effort to match the magazine descriptions of what was beautiful. I saw boys devastated by not making one of the sports teams because they didn't want to disappoint one or both of their parents. It was truly a sobering experience.

I began to ask myself what exactly I thought I could do to change some of the experiences these kids were having. I realized that there were traumas, physical and emotional, that I could not change. But I could provide support to ease a little of that pain. Slowly, I began to see subtle changes in a few of the children. Some of those sad faces turned to smiles and confidence began to build. I learned a lot from those children about caring and kindness, being quiet and listening and persevering through difficult situations. I learned that sometimes the most difficult of personalities were really just scared silly. I learned that bravado and outlandish behaviors sometimes were protective mechanisms. But most of all I discovered the incredible, invincible strength of youth, and their ability to rebound, regroup and try again.

Blessedly, the majority of the young people I encountered were bright, happy and energetic. My care for those children was targeted and brief. But for those troubled by acute or chronic disease, I became a person who could provide some respite, increase their comfort, and help them to reach their full potential. We learned much together, those children and me. Although I taught them how to properly use inhalers, test their blood sugar or stop a nosebleed, they taught me that being a nurse is much more than lots of medical knowledge. It is about seeing the individual for the person they are and helping them to be the best they can be. It's about empathy, not sympathy, optimism instead of skepticism and absolute acceptance. It is about being open-minded and not taking yourself too seriously. It is about proceeding with confidence, including the confidence to ask for help when needed. And most of all, it's about always, always, always having a sense of humor.

School nurses everywhere accomplish this daunting task on a daily basis. It is an honor to be in such magnificent company.

To contact Claire Vey, send an email to cpvey@k12.carr.org.

An Agenda of My Own

By Judith Dorward, RN, MSN

The mandates. These are the things that a school nurse is required, by law, to do. Mandates include vision and hearing screenings and referrals, checks for scoliosis, special education assessments and child abuse reporting. Then there are the other duties: arranging dental care for children with toothaches, counseling troubled teens, advising parents, finding funds for medical services and classroom teaching. The list is never ending.

As I drove to work one late April morning I experienced a familiar feeling. The school year was rapidly coming to a close and I hadn't finished all the mandates. It is an uncomfortable feeling. "Today," I told myself, "I will make a list of all the mandates I haven't finished and then I will start doing them! No interruptions! I will be task-oriented!"

I parked my car in an isolated spot in the parking lot where no teachers would find me. My plan to sneak into my office unnoticed was quickly thwarted as I discovered a ladder directly in front of my door and a large crowd gathered around it. "What's going on?" I asked.

"Manny was vacuuming up there and he found three condoms tied together on the light rod," the campus supervisor said. "He's gone to get some gloves and take them down."

My curiosity was piqued. I climbed the ladder to investigate. Surely there couldn't be condoms—especially not up there. I spotted the objects in question. "I have a Master's Degree in Nursing," I informed the crowd. "And I'm qualified to tell you that these are not condoms. This is a vinyl examination glove." When I'm pressed I sometimes plop ice cubes into a glove and tie the end. It makes a nifty icepack. Someone had tossed his makeshift icepack onto the recessed lighting shelf. Disappointed, the crowd dispersed.

To work I went. *The paper will fly! I'll get organized! I'll make that list and get things done!*

My door opened and in came a student named Nick carrying his bike, out of breath and bloody. He had been in an accident and all of his fingers seem to be dislocated at every joint. After a moment of anxiety, I remembered Nick's congenital joint condition. His joints looked dislocated all the time. One finger, however, was a bloody mess, and obviously broken. I helped Nick clean up, comforted him and called his mother who arrived shortly to take him to the emergency room.

Another student named Emily came in just after Nick with a pass from her teacher. "I have a very sore throat," she said in a voice that revealed a great deal of pain. I looked at her throat and it was about the yuckiest throat I had ever seen. "Let me take your temperature before I call your mother," I said.

Just then, two campus supervisors entered with a student named Rebecca and informed me that she was in labor. Now, it had been many years since I assessed a woman in labor—about twenty-five. I felt her stomach and there was a faint but very real contraction. Rebecca informed me that she was a week overdue. Another contraction came shortly after—they were five minutes apart. Emily, with a sore throat waiting for her mother to pick her up, looked on in horror.

"Where's your mother?" I asked Rebecca.

"She just dropped me off," Rebecca answered. "She won't be at work for an hour."

"Why didn't you tell her you were in labor?"

"I just thought it was something I'd eaten—a little gas," Rebecca said.

I left a message on her mother's answering machine informing her to call me as soon as possible. I then left a message with her doctor's office staff. We continued to time contractions and phoned her boyfriend.

Rebecca's doctor called back and asked, "Is Rebecca in labor? I haven't seen her in over nine months. I didn't know she was pregnant. Maybe you should take her to the emergency room. I don't deliver babies." He offered no help.

Finally, Rebecca's mother called. "I have your daughter here," I said. "She is in labor. She is having contractions five minutes apart. Can you come and get her?"

She burst into tears: "No, no, no, it can't be!"

"Does your mother know about this?" I asked Rebecca.

She looked at the floor.

Emily, the girl with the sore throat, was then greeted by her mother who took her home. The brother of Rebecca's boyfriend, meanwhile, arrived in my health office and took her to the emergency room. The day was going by fast.

Before I had a chance to grab a pen and begin a list of things to do, a student popped in and said, "I have to talk to somebody. Do you have a minute?" Then I got a phone call from a parent who said, "You sent a note that my child needs glasses. I don't have any money or insurance. What can I do?" Another student came in with an abscessed tooth. Next, a psychologist stopped in and said, "I really need you to look at a certain student today." Nick's mother called—he has a cast. Emily's mother called and let me know that Emily had mono.

I called the emergency room and discovered that Rebecca was just seven months pregnant. They gave her medication to stop her premature labor. They also gave her mother something to calm her down.

At 2 p.m. the school day had ended. Everybody left. I found a piece of paper. "LIST," I wrote.

To contact Judith Dorward, send an email to rjdorward@aol.com.

Reflection on a School Nurse's Practice

By Donna Peltier-Saxe, RN, MSN

As I reflect on my job as a school nurse I feel the rewards of this job definitely outweigh the frustrations. There are some days I never get a lunch break or leave my office, and many times I miss a scheduled meeting because of an urgent event that requires my attention. It's hard to plan the day and sometimes frustrating to miss an important meeting with a student's family, the social worker, the special education staff or other faculty. You just never know what you'll be called on to do in this job. Each day brings new situations and new challenges. After working at a large hospital-based healthcare clinic, I was worried that I might get bored—*school nursing certainly isn't boring!*

On an average day at a suburban school of 925 I see 30-40 high school students and on my busiest days I've seen as many as 60 students. I am grateful for the days when I can take time to reflect and try to strategize on what I can do next to help some of my "regular customers" or "frequent flyers." I have several students who need medication administered on a daily basis for chronic illness or conditions such as asthma, diabetes, life-threatening allergies, attention deficit disorders or psycho-emotional disorders. I follow staff members and monitor their blood pressure, advise them when to seek follow-up with their doctor on a multitude of medical problems both acute and chronic and assist staff with any injuries or accidents. I am a resource and referral base internally to resources both within the school as well as to community healthcare providers. On a daily basis anywhere from two to six students visit the health office for lunch. Their conversations are an opportunity to glimpse into their day and see how they're doing. Students share memorable events in their life and discuss their plans and concerns. As I look back on my three years of practice as a school nurse I can say with confidence: "I make a difference." This gives me satisfaction and reaffirms my commitment to continue my professional role as a school nurse.

To provide more insight into why I am committed to school nursing, let me describe some of the highlights of a day in May this year. I saw 33 students over the course of the day.

There were the usual complaints about headaches and there were daily medications to be administered and some complaints about abrasions. Two students with abrasions received in incidents over the weekend had signs of infection that needed to be treated (even the simple presenting complaint of an abrasion can actually be an infected wound). While treating the students I taught them what to expect, how normal wounds heal, and when to seek follow-up in the health office or with their primary care physicians. These are lifelong skills—how to treat wounds and when to seek medical assistance—they will need not only as they head off to college, but throughout life.

A student was ill and not able to tolerate solid foods. The parents of the student were away and the temporary guardian was unavailable to dismiss the student. The student spent the day in the cot room where I made sure he was hydrated and comfortable until his guardian arrived.

Another student complained of cold symptoms with chest pain and discomfort when taking a deep breath. After an assessment I tried to call the parent that the student resides with. After several attempts I had to contact the non-custodial parent to dismiss the student and make sure the student had a doctor's appointment.

Another student required follow-up and dismissal to see the primary care physician. The student complained of difficulty seeing due to an eye that was extremely sore and irritated with inflammation and purulent drainage.

Later, a student came in with a ring on so tight that it restricted circulation. The student was panicking as she experienced swelling, discoloration and loss of sensation in her fingertip. After trying ice, soaps and other methods I had to use a ring cutter to remove the ring. A crisis was resolved and a trip to the emergency room avoided.

Another student returned to follow-up after an emergency room visit the night before. Directions and follow-up instructions that had been given to the student—the importance of taking the medication prescribed as directed, compliance with the dosage times ordered and completing the medication as ordered—were reviewed and reinforced.

A student who complained of neck pain had been diving in the ocean the night before. The hazards of diving head first into unknown depths were reviewed and the risks of devastating injury including paralysis were discussed. Luckily, there was very little evidence of injury. The student agreed to consider jumping feet first into unknown depths in the future.

Two students came into my office to discuss how stressed and overwhelmed they were about completing the work necessary to meet their graduation requirements. It is reassuring to find that students reach out for support when they feel overwhelmed. Offering reassurance, support and seeking other resources within the school to help these students is a major daily challenge.

I've shared this glimpse into just one of my days with the hope of conveying the value and importance, on a daily basis, of the school nurse. The school nurse helps students, families and faculty link to school and community resources as they need them. By sharing a part of one day's events, I hope you begin to understand the impact the school nurse has on whether children have a productive and successful experience at school.

To contact Donna Peltier-Saxe, send an email to dpsaxe@marblehead.com

The ABCs of World Peace

By Kathy Borniger, RN

When I started my job almost nine years ago I was the first registered nurse my school had employed. I'm sure anyone who has been in this position can relate to the many challenges associated with not only being the new kid on the block, but also the *different* kid on the block. While I certainly felt welcomed and valued most of the time, it seemed that I was often defining my job and boundaries in areas where my profession required me to do so. I heard a lot of statements such as "we didn't used to have to do it that way" or "why can't you just give this pill (which was unmarked and in a baggie) to my child if I tell you to?"

Many hours were spent creating new files and updating old ones. At times the task at hand seemed too great, and I questioned my sanity for taking over and trying to improve upon the health office. I talked to myself a lot in those days, wondering aloud, "What am I thinking? This is too difficult." I felt that I would never be organized enough to have a proper health room that complied not only with state and professional guidelines but also with what I thought the job should entail. On top of reception and attendance duties, I was seeing at least 40 students a day. I was overwhelmed.

I began to practice saying, "Would you like fries with that order?" I had pretty much accepted that I was a failure and that my future was in fast food. Paranoia was my pal.

And then it dawned on me. A statement from the mouths of babes caught up with me one day that I think every person, especially adults, can learn from. I most often hear this statement from the little ones—the 225 kids in kindergarten through second grade. They come into the health room from recess with a bump or an abrasion, very dirty and disheveled and sometimes in tears. When I ask them how the injury occurred, they almost always reply, "My friend did it, but didn't mean to."

Amazing! I think we may have the answer to world peace here. If we learn to give the benefit of the doubt to people who hurt us in some way, real or perceived, maybe there wouldn't be so much pain and suffering in our world.

I reevaluated my priorities and concentrated on how I could make a difference in the life of a child. I try to keep that same thought every morning when I unlock the door to my office and turn on the lights. What a privilege it is to be the school nurse.

I've already decided that if I ever write a book about my experiences, I'll entitle it "But My Friend Didn't Mean To..."

To contact Kathy Borniger, send an email to kborniger@yahoo.com.

Is This Job Rewarding?

By Jaime Estrada, MSN

While on a job interview to apply for a school nursing position, I asked, "What is rewarding about this job?" I was a labor and delivery nurse and thought everything would pale in comparison to bringing a new life into this world. I was told how rewarding it is to help a struggling student get glasses or assist a family with resources. I wasn't convinced until I experienced this first hand.

During my first year as a school nurse I was asked to make a home visit to a family with children who had been sick and out of school for a week. When I knocked on the door, I was surprised to see the mother and children as bright as pumpkins. I was sure they had hepatitis, yet they had not been seen by a doctor. When I asked her why she had not sought medical attention, she quite frankly informed me that she could either put food on the table or go to the doctor's office, and asked what choice I would make if I were in her shoes. I was shocked by this response and called public health to treat the family. This was a real eye-opener and a great experience as it taught me that not all people have access to healthcare.

Another rewarding episode occurred as a result of my giving a hearing screening to a kindergartener. She failed numerous attempts at passing the screening, prompting me to call her mother. When I spoke with her, she cried and thanked me. She had suspected something was wrong even though her child had passed her hearing screenings at the doctor's office. The student had been struggling in school and was extremely withdrawn. Once she got her hearing aides, she blossomed.

Indeed, it wasn't long before I was convinced that school nursing is one of the most rewarding jobs available.

To contact Jaime Estrada, send an email to jestrada@cvesd.k12.ca.us.

Ten Years of School Nursing

By Barbara Shannon Davidson, RN, BSN, CSN

The start of 2003 marked ten years since I began my career as a nurse for Chicago Public Schools. As I reflect upon the most meaningful events during those days, I can see the faces of many children whose lives I was able to touch.

When a student was murdered by his uncle who committed suicide, I counseled a number of students who were trying to make sense of such a meaningless tragedy. I explained leukemia to an eighth grade class so they could support a classmate with the condition. I worked with a sexually abused sixth grade girl who could not stop wetting herself at school. I worked with a pregnant thirteen-year-old who was too frightened to tell her mother. A five-year-old boy who was diagnosed with diabetes initially did not want to live, but I was able to counsel him and help him see a better future for himself than he had imagined. I witnessed a valiant mother of two boys, both with hemophilia, who did everything in her power to normalize their school experience. I worked to find proper placement for a five-year-old girl that was blind, cognitively delayed and hypotonic. I worked with a twelve-year-old who had asthma and often cried because other students made fun of her condition.

And in the midst of working with children who faced so much adversity, there were many triumphs. Although I cannot recall each success story from my ten years of school nursing, there are a few that have stuck out. I mainstreamed a five-year-old with spina bifida who is now a freshman at the best college prep school in the state of Illinois. I also worked with a student who was initially medically noncompliant in his treatment for ADHD but improved with proper medication. I helped a thirteen-year-old boy recover from post traumatic stress syndrome after witnessing a murder. His grateful mother called to say that I changed her son's life.

Many other students have touched my life. While their adversity may have been less severe, every one of them was important. I am grateful to have been a part of these children's lives. I was as educated by them as they were by me. Their presence in my life has been true witness to what each of us can offer to others.

Teeth Phobia

By Lisa Formby, RN

Surprisingly, as a four year veteran at a high school with more than 1,200 students, nothing had yet occurred beyond the usual: diabetic and asthma emergencies, cuts, bangs and sprains. With only a week of school left, I felt I was on the downhill slide. I could not have been more wrong.

I was sitting in my office working on reports when one of the assistant principals called for me to go to another building on campus where a student had several teeth knocked out. We hustled to the building to find that the teacher had sent the student to the main office. I asked if the teeth were knocked totally out or broken off. The teachers had no idea; they hadn't found the teeth yet. I searched the room where the incident occurred and immediately spotted the teeth. There were three of them, each about an inch in length. It was no wonder the teachers couldn't find them, they were looking for "little" teeth.

I picked them up, ran to the home-economics department and dropped the teeth in milk. I then went back to the main office and examined the student. The front three bottom teeth were knocked out and there didn't appear to be any damage to the gums. We then went through the regular process of contacting the student's parents and dentist.

When I spoke with the dentist, he asked if I had found the teeth. I told him yes and that they were in milk—I was very proud of myself for remembering to put them in milk. He said, "Well, the milk is okay, but the mouth is the best place for them to be. Do you think that you can put them back in his mouth?"

Now, you have to understand, I may be a nurse but I don't do teeth. My children have lost about thirty teeth between them, and I have *never* pulled a single one. I just don't do teeth. I informed the dentist of this, but he was persistent in asking me to at least try.

I put my gloves on, got the teeth out of the milk, took a deep breath and reinserted the teeth. I can tell you that no one was as shocked as I was that I was able to do that.

Hopefully, by my overcoming my phobia when it comes to teeth, this fourteen-year-old will grow old with his three front teeth in place.

This is my Daughter

By Missy Mohler, RN, BSN

During recess at an elementary school, I was beckoned to the playground where a girl had fallen from the very top of a slide and landed on her back. She complained of having back and neck pain along with tingling in her legs. I immediately sent a teacher to call 911 and stabilized the back and neck of this terrified, crying kindergartner to the best of my ability on a bed of mulch.

In minutes, the squad arrived; all the while I was focusing on this young lady. As the medics walked toward us, I began to rattle off my usual report which included her name, age, and so on. About halfway through my report the medic looked at me and said, "This is my daughter!"

He was terrified and I felt terrible that I didn't make the connection. If I had looked at his face, I would have realized immediately. During my career I had worked in an emergency room and was fully aware that this is the greatest fear for emergency workers that are parents.

Her father and another medic transported her to the hospital for evaluation. She was later diagnosed with only a muscle strain and bruising. A few days later, the little girl arrived at my high school office with her mother to present me with a flower and a homemade thank you card.

If you would like to contact Missy Mohler, send an email to mmohler@loganhocking.k12.oh.us.

Bloody Footprints

By Lori Matz, RN, MSN, CSN

On the frantic first day of school in my urban, socio-economically deprived, elementary school, chaos reigns as children and parents mill about looking for classroom assignments. The phone rings and student records are scattered about in my office. Parents stop by to arrange for medication for their children and to drop off forms. In the midst of all this activity, a custodian stuck his head in my door and alerted me to the fact that bloody footprints were discovered in the upper hallway.

I could only hope that he was mistaken as I continued to field questions and take phone calls. About ten minutes later, John, a second grade student, was brought to my office and said to be the source of the mysterious footprints. When I examined the soles of his feet, I realized that John was indeed the source. The soles of his sneakers were worn through with just a few strands of rubber holding the sides together. After questioning, John admitted to stepping on broken glass on the way to school and cutting his feet. He went on to say that his parents were aware of the condition of his shoes.

I attempted to phone John's home without success—phone service had been disconnected. While washing the dirt and blood from the soles of John's feet, I discovered a few remaining pieces of glass, which I removed. I applied antibiotic ointment and bandaged his feet while the confusion of the first day of school swirled around me. As I can't leave the nurse's office unattended, I appealed to the school principal for assistance. The principal immediately dropped the five tasks he was handling and drove to the nearest shoe store. He returned shortly with a new pair of sneakers and several pairs of socks. Wearing his new shoes and socks, John was ready to return to his classroom with instructions to return the next day and have his feet re-examined.

John returned every morning for the next four days and had his feet inspected, cleansed and re-bandaged. Miraculously, he did not develop an infection or any other residual problems. During the entire course of the week, John's parents never responded to written messages or expressed any interest or gratitude regarding John's situation.

The crisis had been resolved to the best of my ability. I looked forward to the remainder of the school year and the challenges that I face as a school nurse on a daily basis.

Just a Question

By Carol T. Kasper, RN, BSN

She was just a little girl in second grade. She walked into the health room with that proverbial "tummy ache." After assessing that no other symptoms were present, she lay resting quietly in a corner of the health room.

She watched as I cared for child after child. In my busy health room, seeing forty to fifty students a day is not unusual. Through my office walked a little boy who just lost a tooth, a child with a scraped knee and a girl with a sore throat, fever and stomach ache who I was to send home with a recommendation to be tested for a strep infection.

After a little while, I asked the little girl with a stomach ache if she felt well enough to return to class. She answered, "Yes, but can I ask you something first?"

"Sure," I said.

"What's it like being a nurse?" she asked.

My mind started to race. Here was an opportunity to make a difference. I had just a moment to respond and catch this child's interest in an age appropriate way. What to say?

"Well, it's really great," I said. "You get to help people every day and you can work in lots of different places—a hospital, a doctor's office, a school."

"Like you." she responded.

"Yes, like me," I said.

As she was walking out the door she said, "I want to be a nurse someday."

"That's terrific," I said, hoping that this was the sincere response of the child. I watched her go, wondering if I could do more to nurture this seed that I hoped had been planted.

I realized that I could only continue on, doing my job, answering questions, hopefully creating that spark of interest in nursing for one child. I could not dwell on this for long, however, as a first grader had just come in. I turned and smiled, ready for anything.

"What can I do for you?"

To contact Carol Kasper, send an email to LORAC3758@aol.com.

A Home Away From Home

By Gladys M. Brown, RN

For many years I took care of pre-operative and post-operative patients, worked in obstetrics, took care of patients in traction and more. Now I'm working with young adults who are merging into our vast society seeking careers and entering into their world of independence. I work in a student health center at a university where it seems I can look forward to a different experience almost every day.

Students come to this university from all over the world and the excitement generated from being independent for the first time can prove to be overwhelming. The university sends out pre-enrollment packets to people interested in attending and it seems as if some of them never even open the packet. Students arrive unprepared and make enrollment very unpleasant. Our appointment book fills quickly with irritated students needing physicals.

"Ma'am, I forgot to bring the rest of my records. They're back in Philly. Can you call my doctor?" I stood there and thought, *I know you didn't just say what I thought you said*. He turned on his cellular phone and made a long distance call home.

Some parents bring their children to school and try to resolve all enrollment issues before making the drive back home. One mother approached me when it was close to quitting time and said, "I know we don't have an appointment, but can you please give my son a physical so he can get enrolled today? Please?"

"Lady, I am so tired," I answered. "I just don't think we can take anymore walk-ins today."

"If you do this for me, I'll buy you a pop."

"Well, I am a little thirsty," I said, knowing the importance of first impressions.

That old statement about first impressions rings true. Two new students came to the clinic seemingly a bit leery in the presence of strangers. They lashed out for no reason and, instead of lashing back, I gritted my teeth and put forth my best smile. I think my smile threw them into shock—they apologized.

Students go through an adjustment period when leaving home for the first time. They don't have their mom and dad around to tell them what to do, and keeping late hours and trying to make early classes proves to be quite a chore. This causes an overflow of minor complaints. The student thought process is: *I'll go see the doctor—then I can tell my instructor I was sick.*

One young lady arrived at the clinic claiming to have asthma. I've had experience with bronchial asthma, so I can't be fooled. The student whispered, but other than that, there was no wheezing, shortness of breath or dyspnea. I realized that the young lady most likely had a problem, but it sure wasn't asthma.

A young man came to see me with a headache and upset stomach and said he was having trouble sleeping at night. I realized he was truly sincere when he muttered, "I'm just so far away from home. I need my mom." After we decided the best thing for him was to go home and take a nap, I could see the tension easing. The next day he stopped by and let me know he was better.

No two days at the health clinic are alike which makes my job both challenging and interesting. Perhaps the most peculiar episode I've experienced here was when a student needed me to fill out medical documentation for him. After filling out the form and returning it to him, he said, "You wrote down my grandfather's name instead of mine." He had not mentioned his grandfather's name and I, of course, had no idea what his grandfather's name was. I don't know what kind of psychic connection we made that day, but it's one I will always remember.

Later, a young man stopped by my office to turn in some medical records. "The environment here is so cheerful," he said. "It's different than some places I've been." Comments like that help me make it through the day.

There is a song in my heart: "If I can help somebody along the way, then my nursing is not in vain."

To contact Gladys Brown, send an email to gmbrown44@yahoo.com.

VI

Humorous Stories

"Children are wonderful and provide an innocent array of behaviors that keep us guessing everyday."

—Jeffrey D. Carl, RN

Birthday Boy

By Sandy Hearn, LVN

Lunch was over and the elementary students were at recess. The door swung open to the nurse's office and in marched two little kindergarten boys. One of the boys was crying and holding his hands up in the air revealing two little scraped palms. On his head he wore a colorfully decorated party crown with his name printed in large letters on the front.

"Zachary knocked me down and ran over me," he sobbed. "I hurt my hands and my legs. I can't believe he did this to me on my birthday! I just can't believe he did it on my *BIRTHDAY!*"

While cleaning and dressing his minor (but very significant to a kindergartner) wounds, I turned my attention to the little aggressor.

"Zachary, that is not how we treat our friends," I sternly reminded. "What do you say to him?"

Zachary turned to the birthday boy and sheepishly replied, "Sorry. I didn't see your hat."

If you would like to contact Sandra Hearn, send an email to sandra.hearn@leanderisd.org.

The Class Pet

By Charlene Hostetler, RN

Upon arriving to school I received a call to hurry upstairs to one of the science rooms. I walked in to find a young seventh grade boy with his hand locked in a six foot boa constrictor's mouth (the class pet). Apparently, the child was feeding the snake, and as he put his hand in the cage the snake thought it was a mouse and bit down.

The science teacher was desperately trying to get the child's hand released who screamed as the teacher tried to open the snake's mouth. The school administrators soon arrived stunned at what they saw. Despite great efforts, no one could unlock the mouth of the snake.

I stayed with the frantic student and helped calm him while the snake was rubbing against my arm. Amazingly, my focus remained on the child and I truly forgot about the snake on my arm (I am not a fan of snakes). Meanwhile, the teacher made use of a pen to roll back on the snake's jaw, gradually releasing the bite.

We eventually did get the snake to release the child's hand and the incident ended on a happy note. The child was seen in the ER, was treated for the bite and recovered without complications. While the student was previously rather unknown among his classmates, he became a celebrity for the rest of the year. As for the snake, it was carted away by animal control.

The teacher and I were shaken, but what a story we had to tell for many years to come.

If you would like to contact Charlene Hostetler, send an email to charharmony@aol.com.

Hearing Problems

By Tammy Wollbrinck, RN

One of my duties as an itinerant school nurse was to plan, organize, and participate in the Mass Vision and Hearing Screening held yearly at my elementary schools. My second year in this position, I was thrilled by how smoothly the entire process was running. Students were quietly moving from one testing station to the next and we were completing the screenings efficiently and rapidly. Therefore, I was not surprised when one of my kindergartners came up to me and said, "It sure is quiet in here, isn't it, Nurse Tammy?"

I smiled and agreed with him. What confused me was his next comment, "I'm sorry that it is not going very good for you." When I asked why he thought things were not going well, he looked at me with his big, sad, brown eyes and replied, "Teacher says this was supposed to be a mass *screaming*, and nobody is doing what they were supposed to do."

If you would like to contact Tammy Wolbrinck, send an email to tammyw@rangevu.aps.k12.co.us.

The Power of Suggestion

By Mary Currie, RN, BSN

Recently I was asked how my current job as a high school nurse differs from elementary school nursing—where I had started out many years ago. What popped into my head was "psych" nursing. The added element of trying to read minds is much more evident at high school than at elementary school.

A situation that called for "psych" nursing happened not long ago when a student came to my office complaining of a headache between first and second periods. When I questioned her, the student went on to say that she felt pain behind her left eye and thought it might be an aneurysm. I advised her to rest, offered her a cold compress and, after several minutes, she returned to class saying she felt much better. As the day went on, I had two similar situations where a student used the "A" word to describe what they thought they might be experiencing.

Towards the end of the day, as I was picking up my mail in the front office, I mentioned that several students were having bad headaches occurring mainly behind the left eye. I went on to say how odd it was that they were thinking the cause might be an aneurysm. I was stumped and asked if there was a drastic pollen count or humidity change. To my dismay, one of the teachers stated, "Oh, that exact scenario was on an ER rerun last night."

No wonder, I thought, *if I could only get access to the night's television scripts, I'd have an idea of what ailments to expect the next day.*

If you would like to contact Mary Currie, send an email to mcurrie@forsyth.k12.ga.us.

Chicken in Crisis

By Dena Weeks, LVN

It now seems that my duties include chicken care. Our multi-age class of first and second graders hatched two chicks as their class project. One morning in May, one of the baby chicks seemed to be choking and the teacher asked if I knew how to give the Heimlich Maneuver to chickens. I explained that I could make a very good "chicken 'n dumplings," but I usually take care of children (my sincerest apologies for such a horrible, thoughtless statement. I have grown to love Fluffy and will never think about him/her with dumplings again).

Looking at the distressed baby bird wasn't as difficult as facing a room full of seven-year-old eyes pleading, "Help our Fluffy." The ugly, brown, speckled bird staggered around its cage gagging and apparently trying to gasp for breath. My heart ached to see such helplessness but I didn't know anything about treating chickens. With the principal's instruction, I took the baby to the nearest animal hospital.

The first hospital I went to said they "don't do birds" and sent me to the emergency hospital across town. Of course, on this particular day the doctor was not in and I was sent to a rural veterinary clinic several miles outside of town. It seemed that the doctor at this clinic was especially fond of chickens as his clinic actually had a rehabilitation program for birds. Yes, you understand correctly: Chicken Rehab. It's what us folks in the country consider an important endeavor. All chickens should be well adjusted and able to function in society.

By the time Fluffy and I reached this chicken-friendly hospital, he/she had been sliding around the box in the car for a while and had stopped gagging. In fact, Fluffy was chirping as usual.

The staff at the "chicken friendly" animal hospital was very kind and understanding. The animal nurse picked up the chick and gave him/her kisses and praised him/her when he/she went pooh-pooh. My choices were to sign a release of the animal to the rehab program (the chick would not be returned) or pay a great deal of money and take the chance that something could happen to it later. I chose the former and felt secure knowing that Fluffy was loved and had a super chance of living happily ever after.

Laugh, but it is a true story. And the school nurse is a hero to the kids in the multi-age class.

If you would like to contact Dena Weeks, send an email to dgweeks@kellerisd.net.

Now With Both Eyes

By Jeffrey D. Carl, RN

I have been a school nurse for 10 years with the Department of Defense Dependents Schools overseas. I have worked at elementary schools, high schools and everything in-between. I have done STD counseling and have been a boo-boo fixer. I have seen the gambit, but nothing beats this one.

I was doing my annual health screenings at a 750-student K-5 school. I always do the exact same thing with each student during vision screenings so that I know where I am and never get lost while screening. I screen fifth graders first then move downward as my skills are increasingly more challenged respective to the age of the students.

I finally got to the first graders and did my usual screening procedure. One by one, I handed each student a paddle to cover their eye and said, "Cover your right eye with the paddle and read the chart, please... Now cover your left eye and read line number five, please... Now both eyes, please."

The first few students passed through without incident. Approximately the fifth student I screened, however, was doing fine until I said, "now both eyes." He took the paddle and passed it back and forth over each eye attempting to cover both of his eyes. He then set the paddle down and proceeded to cover both of his eyes with his hands.

I was completely overwhelmed with laughter and could not even bring myself to ask him how he could read the chart with both eyes covered. The funniest thing is, this happened about fifty more times, each time provoking uncontrollable laughter. As the day continued, I actually began to very carefully ask each student to read the chart in the same manner to see if they would cover both eyes.

I had to share this with my colleagues, so I positioned the students near a window where they could be seen taking the test. Much to the amusement of the principal and many others, they repeated the same behavior over and over again.

Children are wonderful and provide an innocent array of behaviors that keep us guessing everyday.

If you would like to contact Jeffrey Carl, send an email to jeffrey_carl@eu.odedodea.edu.

Healing Power

By Sue Lang, RN, MPH

As a school nurse serving the special education population (students with severe and multiple handicapping conditions) for the past fourteen years, I experience special situations virtually everyday that make me very proud to be in this position.

In addition to my special education responsibilities, I travel 80 miles to a small K-8 (regular education) school located in a remote desert area. There are approximately 50 students in the entire school and I visit them on a monthly basis. It is from this assignment that I share the following story.

A few years ago, during a routine vision test, I referred a second grader named Adrian for further evaluation because he failed the screening. At the end of the school year, the principal invited me to attend the school's promotion ceremony. To my surprise and shock, a portion of the program was set aside to honor the school nurse! One by one, each student came up and handed me a special card or drawing made especially for this occasion (artwork that I treasure to this day). As Adrian approached, now sporting a good-looking pair of glasses, he said, out loud, "Thank you, Miss Sue. For letting me see."

Code Zebra

By Anne M. Biddle, RN, BSN

One Monday morning rolled around last winter and along came a litany of colds, sore throats and coughs into my nurse's office. Then came Steve. He signed into my daily log, sat down, and gave me a sheepish look.

"What's wrong, Steve?" I asked. Out of his pocket came a piece of paper with one word written on it: ZEBRA. This was the pre-agreed code for: *Something is wrong but I don't want to embarrass this student. Please investigate*. The teachers in my small suburban school are great about communicating and collaborating. Here was a classic example.

When I looked at Steve, I noticed a series of red, uniform size circles on his face and neck. *Ringworm* popped into my head at first glance, but something was oddly different.

After a few moments of questioning him, Steve pulled something out of his pocket with the same sheepish look back on his face. It was a circular suction cup. I thought, *what could this have to do with his problem?*

I understood clearly! Steve admitted how his nervous habit of pushing the suction circle onto his face and neck had created a new diagnosis: self-induced hickeys!

With the ZEBRA note Steve returned to the teacher and explained his problem was not ringworm at all, just our first ever case of SIHS (Self Induced Hickey Syndrome).

A school nurse never knows what situation will present itself each time a student walks through the health office door. Input from teachers plays a key role in helping figure out what is going on with students—especially when there is more than meets the eye.

If you would like to contact Anne Biddle, send an email to annebiddle@comcast.net.

The Eternal Battle

By Jody Lowry, RN, BSN

It was December and as any school nurse worth her weight in lice combs knows, lice are alive and well in Florida! We traditionally work incessantly fighting the eternal "battle of the louse."

It was a particularly challenging week as the children were very excited about the upcoming Christmas break. Teachers were counting the days until their break and we were checking heads, calling parents and dealing with the ancient lice battle!

A large number of students were consistently leaving school for lice treatment only to come back with them two weeks later. In an effort to fix the problem, we counseled parents, educated teachers and even disposed of pillows in the media center. Still, we could not find the real culprit!

Amid our lice situation I was also taking photos of students for a project that was intended to show the joys of life at elementary school. The day before Christmas break, a young boy entered to have his picture taken who happened to come from a class enduring a particularly potent lice outbreak. I took a picture of the child who smiled ear to ear while wearing a reindeer hat from his classroom. The boy explained that his teacher allowed all students to "take turns" wearing the hat!

Our dilemma was solved with that little bit of information!

If you would like to contact Jody Lowry, send an email to joan_lowry@doh.state.fl.us.

The Mysterious Twitch

By Michael J. Murphy, RN, CSN

While working in an elementary school I was approached by a very conscientious kindergarten teacher who was concerned because one of her female students had developed a jerky twitch in one of her arms. Through a glass window in the classroom door, I observed the five-year-old student thoroughly enjoying her surroundings (she was bouncing off the walls).

Once settled down to a series of activities of reading and coloring with crayons, I did notice jerking motions. The motion was an erratic, full extension of the upper extremities, sometimes unilaterally and other times bilaterally, with no apparent pattern. Following a 15-20 minute observation, I smiled and returned to my office.

At the end of the period the kindergarten teacher reappeared in my office inquiring about the child's condition. She was truly concerned about this new development. I couldn't help but smile when I instructed her to simply roll up the child's sleeves prior to hands-on activities.

Many school nurses work in a setting where the tension and stress levels are considerably high. A situation such as this one just brings a smile to one's face.

If you would like to contact Michael Murphy, send an email to mmurphy@wcasd.k12.pa.us.

When Animals Attack

By Diane Stevenson, RN

In my experience as a school nurse I have been particularly amazed by incidents where students have clashed with wild animals.

I took care of a seventh grade student several years ago who arrived at school with a scratched face and skinned arms and legs, not to mention a terrible case of impetigo. When I asked him what happened, he said that he ran into a skunk while riding his bike and fell to the pavement. He had to be excluded from school until he saw a physician for medication. We didn't know whether to believe his story, but as time went on, parents confirmed that he did in fact hit a skunk while riding his bike.

I also took care of a fourth grade student who came into school after suffering a bite from a beaver. While it was hard to believe that he was actually able to get close enough to a beaver to be bitten, I nevertheless sent him to a physician for treatment.

While we do live in a semi-rural area, incidents like this are nevertheless hard to believe.

Out of the Mouths of Babes

By Donna L. Gross, RN

During one fall season of my career as a school nurse we shared our campus with a nearby school that was undergoing construction and therefore had an extra nurse on campus. During this time, the other nurse and I would rotate every day between working in my office and running screenings for hearing and vision.

One morning, while I was in my office, Jake came in to see me. Jake was a sweet first grader whose smile could reach right inside your heart. He said, "I need some more of that stuff."

"Of course," I replied. "What stuff?"

"You know," replied Jake, "the stuff the lady gave me yesterday."

"What did she give it to you for Jake?" I asked.

"For my Kangaroo Sore," answered Jake in a very matter of fact tone.

After a moment of silence, while I digested what he had said, it occurred to me that he meant to say canker sore!

He was so serious that I didn't dare correct him. I just gave him his ointment for his lip and sent him on his way. Of course, this story has provided many people with a good laugh on an otherwise dreary day.

If you would like to contact Donna Gross, send an email to. dgross@mail.gesd.k12.az.us.

1000 Degrees

By Rebecca M. Boutwell, RN, BSN

One early fall morning a first grade boy came into the health office reporting that he did not feel well. I had just arrived at work and was reaching for my thermometer when he asked, "Can your temperature ever be 1000?"

"Oh no," I replied as I placed the thermometer in his mouth. "That would be too hot for the human body to handle. Temperatures never get anywhere close to that high."

Just then the thermometer beeped. He took it out and exclaimed, "Look Nurse Becky, my temperature is 1000!"

In confusion, I took the thermometer out of his hand and smiled. It read: 100.0.

I am Not!

By Trish Green, RN

Not long ago I was color-screening my kindergarten boys. A diminutive, chocolate-skinned boy failed. When I asked him if he knew that he was color blind, he indignantly said, "I am not! My father says I'm half Spanish and half black."

Lessons Learned:

Reflecting on the Daily Joys and Challenges of Elementary School Nursing

By Kathy Noll, RN

Lessons Learned:

- Creative ways to eat lunch in stages
- Frequent flyers never seem to get our message to stay in class
- Scab-picking is a learned art perfected in elementary school
- The delicate process of ongoing hygiene teaching
- Clean is a relative term
- Despite our best ongoing efforts, some required paperwork is never returned
- There is always a new list to be made
- Being thankful for the end of recess
- Rashes are impossible to diagnose over the phone and only appear upon arrival at school
- The large volume of vomiting at an elementary school and the alternative use of waste cans
- Many techniques for calming angry parents
- The comfort that a kind word and Band-Aid can bring to a young child
- When using the copy machine, finding those available empty times and not causing a jam at the end of the day
- Why we need to rewash washed clothing
- All those smiling faces that cannot wait to get in the school building in the morning when the bell rings (you will not see this at the secondary level!)
- How to cope with the frustration and challenge of finding the unreachable parent of a sick child
- Head lice keeps our jobs secure and keeps us from scratching our heads at work
- How many times a cup of tea can be reheated before being finished
- The true value of mittens and a warm coat to a child in winter
- The upsetting significant increase of obesity in our schools and the poor nutrition of our students
- The difficulties finding dental care for a child with chronic tooth pain
- The joy and enthusiasm of a kindergartener
- The ease with which we can talk with children about their bodily functions
- How to graciously accept birthday treats and later dispose of them privately
- The excitement over a plastic tooth box
- Always having dry, chapped hands from frequent hand washing
- The challenge of interpreting the finger pointing when using the Snellen E Vision chart
- The reality that a quiet day is a rare and precious gift